ALLERGIC SKIN DISEASES OF DOGS AND CATS

LLOYD M. REEDY, DVM

Diplomate, American College of Veterinary Dermatology; Animal Dermatology Referral Clinic, Dallas, Texas

WILLIAM H. MILLER, JR., DVM

Diplomate, American College of Veterinary Dermatology; Assistant Professor of Medicine, Department of Clinical Sciences, New York State College of Veterinary Medicine, Cornell University, Ithaca, New York.

A SAUNDERS VETERINARY QUICK REFERENCE HANDBOOK

1989

W. B. SAUNDERS COMPANY

Harcourt Brace Jovanovich, Inc.

Philadelphia, London, Toronto, Montreal, Sydney, Tokyo

W. B. SAUNDERS COMPANY
Harcourt Brace Jovanovich, Inc.

The Curtis Center
Independence Square West
Philadelphia, PA 19106

Library of Congress Cataloging-in-Publication Data

Reedy, Lloyd M.

Allergic skin diseases of dogs and cats/
Lloyd M. Reedy, William H. Miller Jr.

p. cm.

1. Allergy in dogs. 2. Allergy in cats. 3. Veterinary dermatology. I. Miller, William H. (William Howard), 1948– . II. Title. SF992.A44R44 1989 636.7′089697—dc19

ISBN 0–7216–2432–4 88–15850

The front cover illustration by Karen Fling, DVM, is an artist's concept of a mast cell degranulating. Circles and triangles are histamine granules and other inflammatory mediators. Indentions in the cell walls are receptor sites and the "Y" shapes are IgE antibodies. When two IgE antibodies are joined by rectangular-shaped antigen (lower left side), the mast cell degranulates, releasing histamine granules and other inflammatory mediators.

Acquisition Editor: Darlene Pedersen
Production Manager: Frank Polizzano
Manuscript Editor: Keryn Lane
Illustration Coordinator: Ken Green
Indexer: Barbara Hodgson

Allergic Skin Diseases of Dogs and Cats ISBN 0–7216–2432–4

Last digit is the print number: 9 8 7 6 5 4 3 2 1

SAUNDERS VETERINARY QUICK REFERENCE HANDBOOKS

Forthcoming

Peiffer: Small Animal Ophthalmology: A Problem-Oriented Approach

Tams: Small Animal Gastroenterology

Brobst, Parry and Foreyt: Veterinary Laboratory Tests

Loar, Rosenthal, and Susaneck: Small Animal Clinical Oncology

Crowe & Kovacic: Veterinary Emergency and Trauma Care

To

Juanita and Kathy

Preface

The primary purpose of this text is to assist the veterinarian in the diagnosis and management of allergic diseases of small animals. It covers those clinical problems that are commonly seen as well as those that are rare. We have attempted to present this material in a clear, direct manner, anticipating questions that occur during decision-making and, hopefully, providing specific information to allow an individualized approach. Didactic material has been kept to a minimum.

The first chapter sets an immunologic foundation for the ensuing clinical material. In the chapters on the various allergic conditions, considerable attention is given to the pathogenesis and methods of diagnosis, as these are crucial to the appropriate management of the condition. Occasional repetitions in various parts of the text have been allowed to ensure a complete presentation with minimal inconvenience for the reader.

Although the methods of diagnosis and treatment presented represent those currently used by most veterinary dermatologists, they often vary, and the reader may be confused sometimes by a contrast of opinions. In these instances, both authors have included their own methods and opinions, but occasionally even the two of us have disagreed. This shows that the practice of veterinary allergy is an evolving admixture of science and art.

The generous and unstinting help of many people made this text possible. First, we would both like to thank the authors of the numerous texts and periodicals that we have consulted for additional information. Veterinary colleagues, too numerous to name, provided encouragement through continued referral of interesting cases. Without their support, plus the cooperation of many wonderful pet owners, this book could not exist. Also, we should not fail to mention our furry patients that allowed us, hopefully, to do more than merely scratch the surface.

We are especially grateful to our wives, Juanita and Kathy, for their patience and understanding while we were sequestered away for days and nights plus weekends. From the beginning, their support was essential to the successful completion of this manual. We would also like to express appreciation to Sue Hubert for labor above and beyond the call of duty in typing and retyping the manuscript, which lightened our burden considerably. Special thanks to Karen Fling, DVM, for her line drawings and to Darlene Pedersen of W. B. Saunders for her constant encouragement and patience with our numerous delays in completing this manual.

We have enjoyed this undertaking and have found the writing and editing of this manual a personal learning experience. We hope others will find it equally informative.

L. M. Reedy

W. H. Miller, Jr.

Contents

1 The History, Terminology, and Immunology of Allergy

Let us first understand the facts and then we may seek the cause.

Aristotle (384–322 B.C.)

INTRODUCTION

During recent years, veterinarians have become increasingly aware of the importance of allergy in various conditions. Allergic sensitization can affect virtually any tissue in the body and cause a multitude of clinical diseases which vary in their pathogenesis, immunology, and pathology. Consequently, a knowledge of allergy and allergic reactions is important in most areas of veterinary medicine. The correct diagnosis and management of allergic diseases require a thorough knowledge of basic immunologic principles. This first chapter will present some background and the vocabulary necessary to understand the chapters that follow. A brief outline of the immune response and how it applies to allergy is also included. Only basic information is included here; the reader is referred to the supplemental readings for a more complete discussion.

The word allergy (*allos:* other, *ergon:* work) is defined as an altered state of immune reactivity, usually denoting hypersensitivity. The function of the immune system is to protect by distinguishing self from nonself and by eliminating the latter. A functioning immune system is required to prevent attack by internal forces such as tumor cells and autoimmune phenomena and by external forces such as microorganisms and toxic substances. If the normal controls fail, the immune system may not clear noxious substances and may attack harmless materials such as pollens or even self. It would not be too simplistic to suggest that allergy is immunity gone awry.

HISTORY OF ALLERGY

The earliest reference to allergy may be from the Chinese emperor Shen Nung, who in 3000 B.C. forbade pregnant women to eat fish, shrimp, chicken, or horsemeat for fear that these foods might cause ulceration of the skin. The expression "One man's meat is another man's poison" is attributed to Lucretius in the first century B.C. and is believed to have pertained to food allergy. Hippocrates was the first to use the word "asthma" and also may have recognized food allergy by warning in his sixty-fourth aphorism, "It is a bad thing to give milk to persons having headache."

Most of our present knowledge of allergy is based on fundamental observations relating to experimental anaphylaxis in animals. In 1902, Portier and Richet demonstrated that repeated injections of toxic extracts of sea anemone (*Actinaria*) provoked progressively more severe reactions in dogs rather than protection as expected. They coined the word anaphylaxis ("without protection") and theorized that the first injection destroyed any natural resistance the animal might have had to the toxin. Thus, they produced an increased susceptibility rather than immunity. Similar reactions occurred after repeated injections of relatively harmless products such as milk. Anaphylaxis also could be transferred to normal animals by the injection of serum from a sensitized animal. This clearly indicates that some circulating factor confers specific anaphylactic sensitivity.

The erroneous assumption that hay fever in humans was caused by pollen "toxins" prompted early workers to attempt to induce protection against these toxins by immunization. Clinical improvement indicated efficacy of this mode of treatment. The discovery of "blocking antibodies" in the serum of these patients added further support to the usefulness of immunization. In 1923, Coca coined the word atopy (strange disease) to describe a group of human diseases with an inherited predisposition, namely hay fever, asthma, and atopic dermatitis. In spite of the fact that allergic reactions were first discovered in dogs and were extensively studied in other laboratory animals, atopy was erroneously believed to occur only in humans.

Prausnitz and Kustner demonstrated the presence of skin sensitizing antibody (reagin) in the serum of allergic humans by passively transferring it by injection to normal individuals. This important discovery, the P-K test, laid the groundwork for the eventual identification of IgE as reagin or the allergic antibody.

HISTORY OF ALLERGY IN SMALL ANIMALS

As noted previously, immediate hypersensitivity was first described in dogs. Post-mortem examinations of those dogs revealed changes characteristic of anaphylaxis. Since this was artificially induced, there was some doubt that animals other than humans spontaneously developed allergies.

As in humans, the first published, although anecdotal, case reports of canine allergies were to foods. In 1941, Wittich reported on a dog with recurrent seasonal pruritus that coincided with ragweed season. Skin and P-K tests were positive for ragweed and other fall pollens, and the dog was successfully hyposensitized to these pollens. The association of IgE antibodies with canine mast cells was demonstrated in 1973 by Halliwell.

Humans and dogs are not the only species of animal capable of developing spontaneous allergy to aeroallergens. Clinical allergic diseases have been demonstrated in cats, horses, sheep, cows, and a variety of laboratory animals. No doubt allergies exist in all species of animals. Respiratory disease exists in all of these species, and allergy is suspected to play a role in many of these disorders, especially "heaves" in horses. Other allergic diseases such as food hypersensitivity, drug hypersensitivity, insect hypersensitivity, and so on have been documented in many species of animals. Future studies undoubtedly will uncover additional allergic disorders.

DEFINITIONS

Adjuvant is a substance that, when added to an antigen, enhances the immunogenicity of the antigen. Most adjuvants are lipids, bacteria, or insoluble products. Adjuvants heighten the immune response by retarding antigen destruction, by delaying antigen release, or by making the antigen more insoluble. Adjuvants also provoke a local inflammatory response that favors the accumulation of phagocytic and antibody-producing cells.

Allergens are antigens that induce an allergic reaction.

Allergy is an altered state of immune reactivity, usually denoting hypersensitivity. The original meaning of the word was an altered capacity to react. Allergy is an immunologically mediated process wherein a response is mounted against normally innocuous substances (allergens). Immunity implies protection or decreased reactivity, while allergy implies an increased reactivity.

Anaphylactoid reactions clinically mimic anaphylactic reactions but they are not immunologically mediated. Mast cell degranulation can occur via a wide variety of nonimmunologic mechanisms.

Anaphylaxis is an immediate hypersensitivity reaction that is the result of degranulation of sensitized mast cells following reexposure to an allergen. Anaphylaxis typically is thought of as a systemic hypersensitivity leading to a shock-like state, but it can be localized to one specific area, especially the gastrointestinal tract, nasal mucosa, or skin. Anaphylactic reactions typically are mediated by IgE, but IgG also can play a role.

Antibody is a complex protein that is produced as a result of the introduction of an antigen. It has the ability to combine with the antigen that stimulated its production. The word immunoglobulin also is used.

Antigen is a substance that is capable of inducing a detectable immune response. An antigen also has the ability to react with the specific antibody or sensitized lymphocyte generated by the immune response. Most antigens are organic macromolecules in a colloidal state and are usually proteins. Synthetic polymers of amino acids, polysaccharides, nucleic acids, or lipids also may be antigenic. Most effective antigens have a molecular weight of greater than 10,000 daltons.

Atopy is a genetically determined abnormal state of immediate hypersensitivity. In humans, atopy consists of hay fever, asthma, and atopic dermatitis, while in animals the term is applied to inhalant allergic dermatitis.

Cross-reaction is the reaction of an antibody with an antigen other than the one that induced its formation. Cross-reacting antigens share some common determinant groups. Some grass pollens have similar determinant groups so an individual allergic to one grass may react to certain other grass pollens.

Cytotropic antibody is antibody that can attach to or sensitize cells. Homocytotropic antibodies are those that will fix to tissues of animals within the same species, while heterocytotropic antibodies will fix to tissues of different species.

Determinant groups are individual chemical structures present on the antigen which determine antigenic specificity. The number, type, and nature of the determinant groups determine the immunologic uniqueness of an antigen. Two or more antigenic determinants are necessary to stimulate an immune response. Antigens that share common determinant groups immunologically could be viewed as similar and may cross-react.

Haptens are substances that are not immunogenic but can react with an antibody of appropriate specificity. Haptens are also called incomplete antigens and are low molecular weight, simple chemicals. For a hapten to induce an immune response it must be coupled to a larger carrier molecule, which in itself need not be antigenic. A hapten can be thought of as an antigenic determinant of a particular type.

Immunogenicity is the property of a substance which makes it capable of inducing an immune response. The immunogenicity of an antigen is dependent on the molecular size, solubility, shape, electric charge, and accessibility of its determinant groups.

Immunotherapy describes the process of preventing or diminishing allergic symptoms via modulation of the immune response. Previously, this process was called desensitization, hyposensitization, or "allergy shots."

Intolerance is an exaggerated, nonimmunologic physiologic response to a substance. The term is used to distinguish symptoms caused by an idiosyncrasy or an irritation to a substance from those caused by allergy. Erythromycin-induced vomiting is a good example of drug intolerance.

THE IMMUNE SYSTEM

The immune system is extremely complex and new information about its function and regulation is being added daily. Classically, the immune system has been divided into three separate arms, namely the nonspecific, the humoral, and the cellular. Each of these has various components that can interact, and complex interactions occur between the arms. As can be seen from Figure 1–1, an immunologic reaction does not occur in isolation but can affect all parts of the immune system. A defect in one arm or the interactive control mechanisms will result in disease. The following discussion on the various components of the immune system should allow the reader to better understand allergic disorders.

Immunologic Reactivity

Unless the animal has preformed antibodies or activated cells, an immunologic reaction does not occur immediately with the first exposure to an antigen. Immunologic activation occurs immediately, but there is a lag phase of 7 to 14 days before antibody production or cell sensitization reaches a significant level. Since memory cells are generated during the initial or primary immune response, the response to a reintroduced antigen is much quicker and more marked.

Immune Regulation

Although the various cells of the immune system have independent functions, all the cells of the immune system work in concert. For example, the immune response to a simple staphylococcal infection involves primarily the neutrophil. For optimum neutrophil

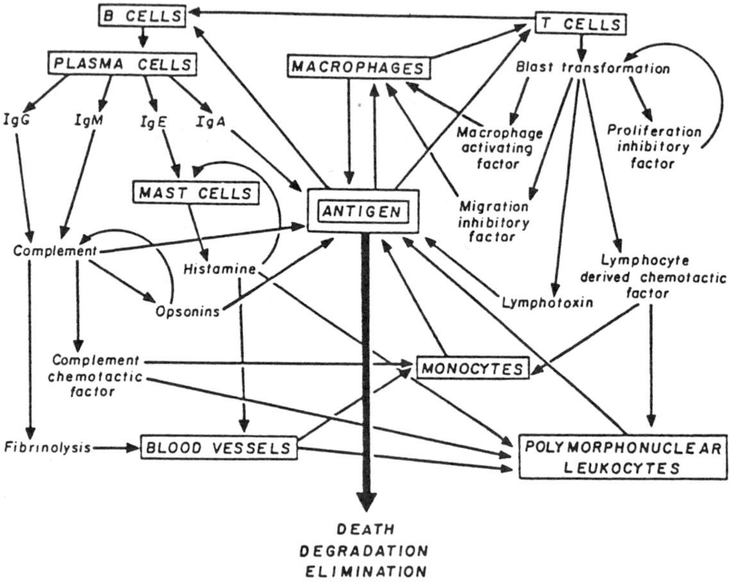

FIGURE 1–1. The immune system—a complex system of interrelated components. The activity of one component often affects others. (Reproduced with permission from Dahl, M.V.: Clinical Immunodermatology, 2nd edition. Copyright © 1988 by Year Book Medical Publishers, Inc., Chicago, p. 2.)

function, chemotactic factors must draw these cells to the area of infection and the bacteria should be opsonized (coated) with antibody or complement or both. For antibody to be produced, B lymphocytes must be activated by helper T cells. These regulatory T cells themselves are activated by macrophages but can be inhibited by suppressor T cells. Figure 1–2 outlines the cellular interactions of the immune system. All of the cells activated contain or produce factors that can potentiate or dampen the immune response. With all these considerations, it is obvious that there is no simple immune response.

The Neutrophil

The neutrophil is a bone marrow–derived cell that migrates into tissues where it is the principal cellular mediator of acute inflammation. The neutrophil plays a central role in the host's defense against infection but is also important in other immunologic reactions.

The neutrophil is the primary phagocytic cell for rapidly dividing

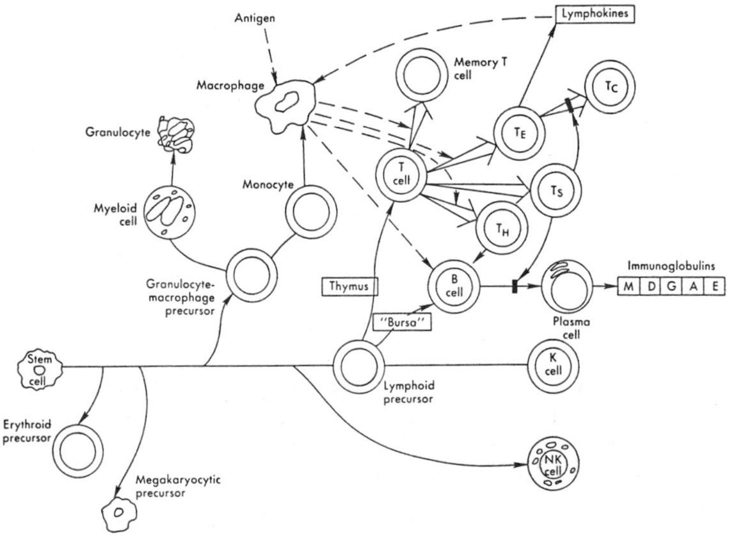

FIGURE 1–2. Outline of cellular interaction in immune system. (Reproduced by permission from Rose, N.R.: Origins of the immune system. *In* Stone, J. (ed): Dermatologic Immunology and Allergy. St. Louis, 1985, The C.V. Mosby Co., p 5.)

organisms such as *Staphylococcus* species, while the macrophage deals more efficiently with facultative or intracellular organisms. For both cell lines, a sequence of locomotion, recognition, ingestion, degranulation, and intracellular killing occurs.

Neutrophil migration is influenced by a variety of chemotactic factors that include histamine, eosinophilic chemotactic factor of anaphylaxis (ECF-A), platelet-activating factor (PAF), neutrophil chemotactic factor (NCF), and leukotriene B_4 (LTB_4) from mast cells; prostaglandins (PG) and leukotrienes (LT) from a variety of cells; $C3_A$, $C5_A$, and $C\overline{567}$ from the complement cascade; kallikrein from the kinin system; plasminogen activator, fibrinopeptides, and fibrin-derived products from the coagulation system; and lymphokines, bacterial products, and immune complexes.

Neutrophils have complement and IgG receptors on their surfaces which mediate the binding of opsonized (antibody- and/or complement-coated) particles to the cell membrane. Small particles are interiorized into a membrane-bound phagosome. Phagocytosis or adherence activates the cell to produce or release reactive oxygen products, leukotrienes, prostaglandins, and enzymes. These agents are released into the phagosome or into the external environment when the adherent particle cannot be ingested. Products released into the fluid space can damage tissues, activate other cells, or initiate the humoral amplification system. Leakage of enzymes from the phagosome into the cell's cytoplasm will result in cell death with the release of all mediators into the extracellular fluid space.

The reactive oxygen products have microbicidal activity but also suppress lymphocyte proliferation and immunoglobulin synthesis and can damage tissues. Neutrophil granules contain acid hydrolases, neutral proteases, and other substances that have antimicrobial activity. The neutral proteases, such as elastase and collagenase, can cause significant tissue damage if they are not inactivated by plasma protease inhibitors. Neutrophil death or secretion of materials from within the cell will amplify the inflammatory response.

The Eosinophil

The eosinophil is a cell typically associated with allergic and parasitic reactions. In the dog and cat with inhalant allergies, the eosinophil is not a prominent cell type. Since eosinophilia is usually modulated by T lymphocytes, the lack of eosinophils in pets could indicate a cell-mediated cause for their allergic disease. Alternatively, the various stimulants for eosinophilia such as ECF-A may not be important in companion animals.

The eosinophil has receptors for complement and IgG on its cell surface and contains granules with proteins and various enzymes. One enzyme, peroxidase, can cause mast cell degranulation and, in combination with hydrogen peroxide and a co-factor, inactivates slow-releasing substance of anaphylaxis (SRS-A).

Although the eosinophil is a phagocytic cell, its primary function in allergic disorders is to modulate the mast cell mediators. Eosinophils have both H_1 and H_2 cell surface receptors for the binding of histamine. H_1 activation augments eosinophil function while the effects of H_2 are inhibitory. In addition to their ability to inactivate SRS-A, eosinophil granules contain histaminase to inactivate histamine, kininase to inactivate kinins, proteins to inactivate heparin, and phospholipase to degrade PAF. Activated eosinophils release leukotrienes and prostaglandins that can modulate the inflammatory response.

The Mast Cell

Mast cells are oval- to spindle-shaped cells with numerous large, intracytoplasmic, basophilic, and metachromatic granules that arise from undifferentiated mesenchymal cells. Mast cells are widely distributed in connective tissues and, in the skin, are prominent around dermal blood vessels. In the dog, 4 to 12 mast cells per high-power field is considered normal, while up to 20 can be found in normal cats. The mast cell is a biologic time bomb loaded with preformed mediators of inflammation and pruritus, which can be

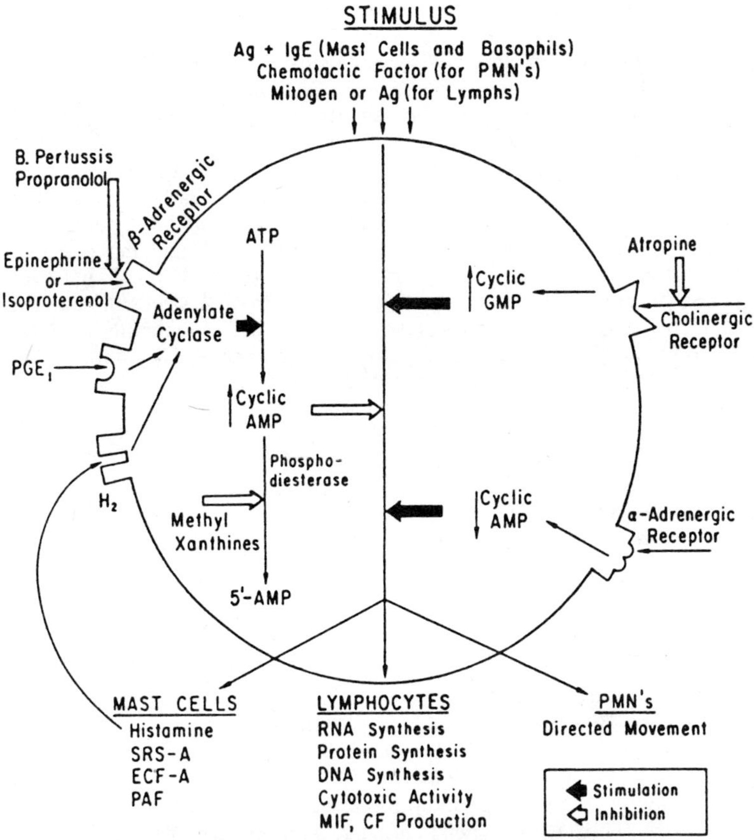

FIGURE 1–3. Diagrammatic representation of pathways by which pharmacologic mediators might act on mast cell, lymphocyte, and PMN leukocyte membrane receptors to alter intracellular cyclic nucleotides, which in turn may either enhance or inhibit the function of those cells. Ag = Antigen; PGE_1 = prostaglandin E_1; SRS-A = slow-reacting substance of anaphylaxis; ECF-A = eosinophil chemotactic factor of anaphylaxis; PAF = platelet-activating factor; MIF = migration inhibition factor; CF = chemotactic factor. (From Hanifin, J.M. and Lobitz, W.C.: Newer concepts of atopic dermatitis. Arch Dermatol 113:663, 1977. Copyright 1977, American Medical Association.)

activated by a variety of substances. Receptors for prostaglandins, histamine (H_2 type), adrenergic and cholinergic agents, and immunoglobulins are found on the mast cell membrane. Stimulation of these receptors alone or in combination activates or stabilizes the cell.

Mast cell activation or degranulation can be caused by the bridging of IgE molecules, anaphylatoxins $C3_A$ and $C5_A$, enzymes, drugs, physical stimuli, and other agents (Fig. 1–3). After stimulation, adenylate cyclase is activated and the phosphorylation of several proteins occurs. Simultaneously, phospholipases, especially phospholipase A_2, are activated which liberate free arachidonic acid and alter membrane fluidity. A transient calcium flux occurs across the membrane which causes the granules to swell and move toward the cell membrane. The granules push the cell membrane from the inside and produce multiple bulges from the cell surface. The perigranular membrane fuses with the cell membrane, and the granule is discharged into the extracellular space. Histamine can be found in the extracellular space within 15 seconds of activation. Aside from containing histamine, mast cells contain a variety of chemotactic factors, enzymes, and proteoglycans and will form mediators from the liberated arachidonic acid.

Histamine is the primary vasoactive mediator released from the mast cell. The effects of histamine are exerted through interactions with the H_1 and H_2 receptors on cell surfaces. In the skin, H_1 activation causes the induction and augmentation of the wheal and flare reaction, increases vascular permeability by causing venular endothelial disconnections, and stimulates the production of prostaglandins. Stimulation of H_2 receptors causes inhibition of lymphocytotoxicity, stimulation of suppressor lymphocytes, inhibition of further mast cell degranulation, and increases in vascular permeability. Pruritus appears to be mediated by the H_1 receptor. Directed and random migration of eosinophils and neutrophils is also affected by histamine. H_1 activity stimulates migration while H_2 activity inhibits it. Histamine and prostaglandin-generating factor of anaphylaxis (PGF-A) cause neighboring cells to produce prostaglandins.

Other vasoactive substances include platelet-activating factor, the leukotrienes, and prostaglandins. These mediators are not preformed but are produced after the mast cell is activated. Leukotriene and prostaglandin synthesis is discussed later.

The mast cell liberates a variety of chemotactic factors that attract inflammatory cells into the area. Histamine, heparin, and proteolytic enzymes from the mast cell cause vasodilation, increases in vascular permeability, and loosening of connective tissues and ground substances, such that the attracted cells can easily enter the area.

Platelet-activating factor (PAF) is an unstored potent lipid that causes the aggregation and activation of platelets. Additionally, PAF augments neutrophil migration, causes neutrophil aggregation, and induces leukotriene synthesis within the neutrophil. PAF causes vasoconstriction and induces vascular permeability.

Eosinophilic chemotactic factor of anaphylaxis (ECF-A) is a preformed factor that attracts and deactivates eosinophils. Other chemotactic mediators stored in or produced by the mast cell include neutrophil chemotactic factor (NCF), T lymphocyte chemotactic factor, B lymphocyte chemotactic factor, and leukotriene LTB_4.

Aside from the vasoactive substances and chemotactants, mast cell granules contain the proteoglycans, heparin, and various enzymes such as tryptase, arylsulfatase, peroxidase, superoxide dismutase, β-hexosaminidase, and β-glucuronidase. Tryptase cleaves C3 to active $C3_A$ and degrades kininogen, which blocks the formation of bradykinin. Heparin is an anticoagulant that works in concert with tryptase to inactivate $C3_A$.

The Basophil

The basophil is a multilobular, bone marrow–derived cell that is motile and capable of phagocytosis. Because of the small numbers of these cells, little information is available about their cellular constituents and function. The basophil often is found in inflammatory reactions involving delayed hypersensitivity and also plays a role in anaphylactic reactions. As with mast cells, basophils have surface receptors for IgE molecules, and bridging of two adjacent molecules may cause degranulation with the release of various chemotactic factors and vasoactive substances, especially histamine. The basophil can be thought of as a circulating mast cell.

THE ARACHIDONIC ACID CASCADE

Essential fatty acids are integral components of cell membranes, and their oxidative products act as local hormone-like regulators of cell function (Fig. 1–4). Dihomo-γ-linolenic, arachidonic, and eicosapentaenoic acids act as precursors of various biologically active lipids (eicosanoids), namely the prostaglandins (PG_S), thromboxanes (TXA_2), hydroxyeicosatetraenoic acids ($HETE_S$), and leukotrienes (LT_S). Arachidonic acid metabolism leads to the formation of the two series of prostaglandins and the four series of leukotrienes.

In cells, arachidonic acid is stored in an esterified state in which it is unavailable for metabolism. Under the action of phospholipase A_2, free arachidonic acid is released and is metabolized by a cyclooxygenase pathway to prostaglandins and by a lipoxygenase pathway to the leukotrienes, LTA_4, LTB_4, LTC_4, LTD_4, and LTE_4. LTA_4 is an unstable intermediate that can be hydrolyzed to LTB_4 or conjugated with glutathione to form LTC_4, LTD_4, and LTE_4. LTC_4,

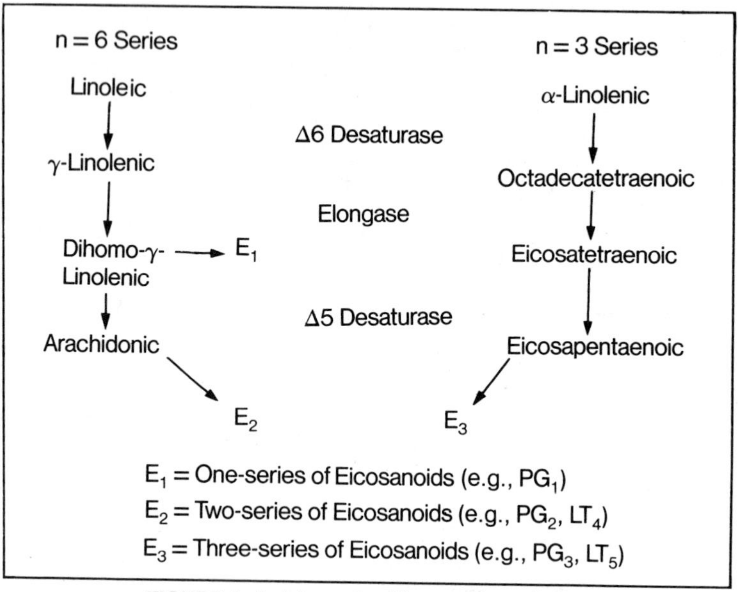

FIGURE 1–4. Schematic of fatty acid metabolism.

LTD_4, and LTE_4 form slow-releasing substances of anaphylaxis (SRS-A).

Prostaglandins cause the alteration of vascular permeability, potentiate the effects of the vasoactive substances, potentiate the sensations of pain and itch, and modulate the immune system. SRS-A increases vascular permeability and enhances prostaglandin production. LTB_4 is a potent chemotactic factor for neutrophils and alters vascular permeability. LTB_4 is also chemotactic for eosinophils and can modify lymphocyte function. Leukotrienes potentiate the effects of the prostaglandins and vice versa and also modulate the immune system in a wide variety of ways.

HUMORAL AMPLIFICATION SYSTEMS

Four separate but integrated serum protein systems affect an animal's immune responsiveness. The complement, coagulation, kinin, and fibrinolytic systems each are composed of a series of proteins, substrates, inhibitors, and enzymes which produce a specific response. Products from one system can activate or modulate another system, so all are related. These systems are dynamic;

proteins must be activated in an orderly, sequential fashion, and undamped activation is prevented by a variety of inhibitors.

The Complement System

The complement cascade is composed of at least 20 chemically and immunologically distinct proteins that interact with each other, with antibodies, and with cell membranes. The complement cascade is the primary humoral mediator of antigen-antibody reactions that result in the formation of products which increase vascular permeability, induce histamine release from mast cells, are chemotactic for polymorphonuclear leukocytes, and are cytotoxic. Complement activation can occur via the classic or alternative pathway.

The classic pathway is activated by the binding of C1 to an appropriate immunologic or nonimmunologic substrate or by the direct attack of trypsin-like enzymes on C1. Immunologic activation occurs when C1 binds to the F_C region of IgG or IgM molecules found in immune complexes or aggregations of immunoglobulins. Nonimmunologic activation occurs when C1 binds to nucleoproteins, staphylococcal protein A, and certain microbial or cell membranes, or by the direct proteolytic effect of trypsin and plasmin on the C1 molecule. The alternative pathway activation typically is independent of immunoglobulins, and stimuli include microbial polysaccharides, lipopolysaccharides, and certain cell membranes. Small amounts of $C3_B$ are constantly produced from the spontaneous hydrolysis of C3. While most of this $C3_B$ remains in the fluid phase, some binds to cell surfaces where it is rapidly inactivated. When $C3_B$ is deposited on the surface of an activator of the alternative pathway, it is protected from inactivation and interacts with other factors to trigger the cascade. The alternative pathway joins the classic pathway at the C5 level.

During complement activation, anaphylatoxins ($C3_A$, $C5_A$, and possibly $C4_A$) are generated, which induce histamine release from mast cells and increase vascular permeability. $C3_A$, $C5_A$, and $C\overline{567}$ are chemotactic for polymorphonuclear leukocytes.

The Coagulation System

Blood clotting involves the formation of a platelet plug and the activation of the clotting cascade, which generates a variety of factors, some of which are important in allergic reactions. Platelet aggregation and activation are under the control of cAMP. They are regulated by products of the cyclooxygenase metabolism of arachidonic acid generated in the endothelial cells of the vessel wall. Thromboxanes (TXA_2) induce low cAMP levels which cause strong aggregation, while prostacyclins (PGI_2) cause increased cAMP levels and inhibit platelet aggregation. TXA_2 also causes local vasoconstriction while PGI_2 causes vasodilation. These two agents work in concert with each other to regulate platelet plug formation.

In the fashion of the complement cascade, there is a series of clotting factors, which is activated sequentially by either an intrinsic or extrinsic method. The intrinsic pathway is activated when factor XII (Hageman factor) is absorbed onto an exposed surface. This binding results in molecular conformation changes which enable factor XII to convert prekallikrein to kallikrein. Kallikrein converts factor XII to its fully active form, factor XII_A, and can also trigger the formation of kinins, plasmin, and factor XI_A. Activated factor XI_A activates factor IX that, in combination with factor VIII, creates factor X_A.

The extrinsic pathway is triggered by tissue thromboplastins that are composed of phospholipids plus a tissue factor. The phospholipids seem to serve as a binding site for clotting factors, while the tissue factor acts as a co-factor for factor VII. Kallikrein and factor XII_A also can activate factor VII. The complex of factor VII, the tissue factor plus calcium, and phospholipids activates factor X.

Once the activated factor X is generated, by either the intrinsic or extrinsic pathway, it will convert prothrombin to thrombin. Thrombin then converts fibrinogen to fibrin. Thrombin can cleave C3 to $C3_A$ and can activate C5. C1 inactivator can inactivate factor XII_A, kallikrein, and factor XI_A.

The Kinin System

Activation of clotting factor XII results in the formation of kallikrein, which cleaves kininogen to kinins, especially bradykinin, and is itself chemotactic for polymorphonuclear leukocytes. Kallikrein also can cleave C5 and convert plasminogen to plasmin, which can activate the alternative complement cascade. Kinins cause vasodilation and increase vascular permeability. Bradykinin can be inactivated by kininases, and its formation can be inhibited by C1 inactivator.

The Fibrinolytic System

The fibrinolytic system is designed to dissolve the fibrin in the hemostatic plug so that the damage can be repaired. Fibrin is digested by the enzyme plasmin derived from its precursor plasminogen.

Plasmin generation can be triggered by factor XII_A, factor XI_A, factor B of the complement system, kallikrein, urokinase, or tissue plasminogen activators from lymphocytes, macrophages, basophils, fibroblasts, or vascular endothelial cells.

Plasmin can activate C1, destroy the C1 inactivator, cleave C3 and C5, and digest fibrinogen and clotting factors XII_A, V, and VIII.

THE MONOCYTE-MACROPHAGE

The monocyte develops from bone marrow precursors but does most of its functional development outside the bone marrow. Cells migrate into tissues where they develop into long-lived macrophages. These mononuclear cells have an important phagocytic function but, more importantly, play a critical role in immune regulation.

As phagocytes, macrophages act as scavengers of cellular debris and inorganic materials and are capable of ingesting infectious agents. Unlike neutrophils, which do not have any energy reserve, macrophages can synthesize new enzymes on demand and thus sustain the phagocytic response. These cells function in a similar fashion as neutrophils in that they migrate in response to chemotactants, adhere via surface immunoglobulin or complement receptors, ingest after cellular activation, and destroy via enzymatic degradation and a respiratory burst that produce reactive oxygen products. Degradative enzymes are stored within granules or within the lysosomal system. Certain organisms such as *Mycobacterium* spp. resist intracellular killing and can multiply protected within the cell. Cell death eventually occurs, releasing organisms and degradative enzymes that damage tissues.

The most crucial role of the macrophage is the regulation of the immune response via antigen processing and the synthesis and secretion of a variety of factors. If an ingested antigen is not completely destroyed, some molecules will persist and will be presented to lymphocytes to initiate an immune response. Since inadequate or excessive antigen presentation can block an immune response, macrophages also regulate the amount of antigen presented. Antigen presentation may involve the complexing of the antigen to the cellular RNA to form a super antigen, or the structure of the antigen may be read by the cell and be encoded into the RNA, which would act as a template for lymphocyte recognition. The antigen activates a T lymphocyte, affecting other lymphocytes.

Activated macrophages synthesize and secrete a variety of enzymes and inflammatory mediators as well as factors that regulate the immune response. Macrophages synthesize the major complement components and a monokine called interleukin 1 (IL_1). Interleukin 1 activates both B and T lymphocytes, is chemotactic for neutrophils, stimulates fibroblasts, increases plasma fibrinogen levels, and causes hepatocytes to produce the acute-phase proteins. Acute-phase proteins include C-reactive protein, serum amyloid A, C3, transferrin, and ceruloplasmin. These proteins probably modulate the immune response so that excessive tissue damage does not occur.

Macrophages also are a source of interferon and endogeneous pyrogens. Endogenous pyrogens stimulate prostaglandin synthesis within the hypothalamus, which has a direct pyrogenic effect. Endogenous pyrogens also induce the synthesis of acute-phase proteins, the proliferation of certain lymphocyte populations, and the degradation of muscle protein. Endogenous pyrogens appear to be similar or identical to IL_1. Macrophages can act as killer cells and may help regulate natural killer cells.

B Lymphocytes

B lymphocytes or B cells are the antibody-secreting cells of the immune system. These cells have immunoglobulins on their surface and possess F_C and complement receptors. The cell-bound antibody molecules function as antigen receptor sites. It is believed that there is one B cell capable of recognizing each unique antigen. B cell activation requires antigen binding plus a signal from the T helper (T_H) cell. Activated cells divide repeatedly, and the offspring differentiate into plasma cells or memory cells.

Memory cells are long-lived, antigen-specific amplifier cells that function in secondary or anamnestic responses. At the first exposure to an antigen, only one or a few B cells can recognize and respond to the antigen. In this initial response, many memory cells are generated. With subsequent re-exposure to the antigen, these multiple memory cells respond, giving a quicker and more intense humoral response.

Plasma cells are the antibody-producing cells; they produce antibodies with the same antigenic specificity as that found on the immunoglobulin bound to the original B cell. Plasma cells can produce different classes of immunoglobulin. The first antibody of an immune response is IgM. As the reaction progresses, plasma cells can switch to IgG or IgE production. These antibodies all retain the same antigen specificity. With antigen removal, B cell activation stops and the plasma cells die. Suppressor T cells (T_S) can inhibit antibody production via interference with B cell activation or by a direct inhibitor effect on the plasma cell.

Antibodies

Antibodies or immunoglobulins are protein molecules synthesized by lymphocytes as antigen receptors or by plasma cells in response to an antigen challenge. Circulating immunoglobulins bind to the antigen that induced their production, hastening antigen destruction. Cytotropic antibodies bind to cells as well as to antigen.

Five major classes of immunoglobulins, namely IgG, IgM, IgA, IgD, and IgE, are recognized. All immunoglobulins have the same basic four polypeptide chain structure consisting of two light and two heavy chains (Fig. 1–5). Each of these chains has a constant and a variable region where the amino acid sequence is either constant or variable. The amino acid sequence in the constant region of the heavy chain determines the class of the antibody. For example, IgG

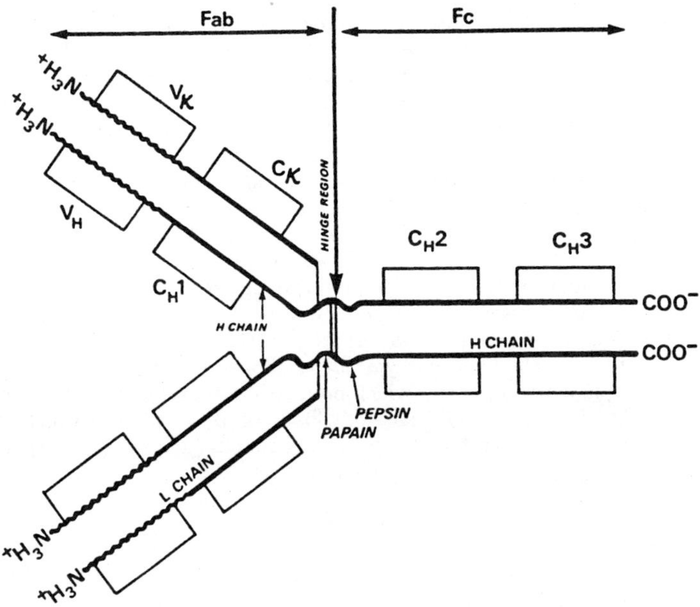

FIGURE 1–5. **A simplified model for an IgG1 (k) human antibody molecule showing the 4-chain basic structure and domains. V indicates variable region; C, the constant region; and the vertical arrow, the hinge region. Thick lines represent H and L chains; thin lines represent disulfide bonds. (Reproduced with permission from Goodman, J.W. and Wang, A.: Immunoglobulins: Structure, diversity, and genetics. *In* Stites, D.P., Stobo, J.D., and Wells, J.V. (eds): Basic and Clinical Immunology (ed 6). Copyright Appleton & Lange, 1987, p 28.)**

has two γ heavy chains while IgE has two ϵ heavy chains. In nature, these chains are folded so that the molecule appears to have six globular units.

Immunoglobulin molecules are divided into the F_{AB} region where antigen binding occurs and the F_C region where cell binding occurs. The F_C region of the IgE molecule has a special segment that facilitates binding to mast cells. IgG and IgM also bind complement in the F_C region. Antigen binding occurs in the variable zone of the F_{AB} region. Although the heavy and light chains each have some individual binding activity, the natural binding site for an antigen involves both chains. Since each basic unit has two F_{AB} regions, it can bind to two antigens.

Antibodies have a unique amino acid sequence in the variable region that enables them to recognize a specific antigen or one very similar to it (cross-reaction). Plasma cells can produce one class of antibody or switch from the production of IgM to IgG, IgA, or IgE. Switching is under genetic control. Genes that code for the amino acid sequence in the variable region remain unchanged, while those that code for the constant region of the heavy chain are replaced. Thus, one plasma cell can produce different classes of antibodies, all with the same antigenic specificity.

IgG is the most abundant antibody and is the basic workhorse of the immune system. IgM molecules are the first antibodies produced in an immune response. The IgM molecule is composed of five basic immunoglobulin structures held together by a joining (J) chain. Each IgM molecule has 10 antigen-binding sites and avidly fixes complement and opsonizes antigens. IgA is thought of as a secretory protective antibody of the respiratory, gastrointestinal, and urogenital tracts. The molecule typically is a dimer in which two basic units are joined by a J chain, which protects it from proteolytic digestion. IgD is a noncirculating antibody found on B cell surfaces which acts as the antigen receptor. IgE is the antibody generated in response to parasitic infections or allergens.

IgE

IgE is a homocytotropic antibody with a molecular weight of approximately 190,000 and a sedimentation coefficient of 8_s. Typical of monomeric immunoglobulins, IgE is composed of four polypeptide chains that are covalently linked by S—S bonds. IgE is found in the fast gamma region of a protein electrophoresis and is heat and acid labile. Heating of IgE to 56° C alters the F_C portion of the molecule. Two F_C antigenic determinants probably exist on canine IgE, and each has a different degree of heat lability. One determinant is very heat labile and can be destroyed within 30 minutes; extended heating is required to destroy the other. Canine and human IgE share some heavy-chain antigenic determinants.

In humans, IgE has the lowest serum concentration due to the highest turnover rate, shortest half-life, and lowest synthesis rate of any immunoglobulin. Metabolic turnover studies in humans have shown that IgE has a total body pool of 0.01 mg/kg (1030), a synthesis rate of 0.004 mg/kg/day (36), a plasma half-life of 2.7 days (21), and a fractional turnover rate of 94.3 percent/day (6.9). For comparison purposes, the mean values for IgG are shown in the parentheses. The fractional turnover rate is the percent of the plasma pool which is catabolized and cleared into the urine per day. In humans, IgE survival is prolonged as the serum levels increase. Apparently, IgE catabolism is associated with its tissue fixation. Tissue-fixed antibody is metabolized more rapidly than plasma antibody. As the serum levels increase, the number of mast cell receptors becomes saturated and much IgE remains unfixed and is metabolized more slowly.

The IgE levels in dogs are much higher than they are in humans, but IgE still is the least concentrated immunoglobulin of the dog. Halliwell has shown that IgE binds only to mast cells (and basophils), but the correlation between serum levels and that bound to the skin is poor. Metabolic turnover studies have not been reported, but, because of similarities in P-K reactivity, the metabolic trends shown in humans probably apply to the dog.

T Lymphocytes

T lymphocytes or T cells comprise most (60 to 80 percent) of the mononuclear cells in the peripheral circulation and greater than 90 percent of the lymphocytes in the lymph channels. T cells can be considered the immunologic surveillance cells of the body. They have surface markers and antigen receptor sites on their cell membranes. There is one T cell or clone thereof for every unique antigen.

Presently, five subpopulations of T cells have been recognized. Regulatory T cells include the helper cell (T_H), the suppressor cell (T_S), and the memory cell. T_H cells are activated by interleukin 1 (IL_1) and are necessary for B cell activation and the switch in antibody synthesis from one class to another. T_S cells produce an inhibitory effect on B cells, plasma cells, and cytotoxic T cells (T_C). A balance between the effects of the T_H and T_S cells regulates the immune response. Memory cells are inactive cells used for an anamnestic response.

The effector arm of the T cell line is the effector T cell (T_E) and the cytotoxic T cell (T_C). The T_C is activated by lymphokinins and is responsible for the killing of cells. Effector T cells produce lymphokines that have a wide variety of action.

Lymphokines

Lymphokines are soluble mediators produced by lymphocytes which affect a variety of cells. A lymphokine can have one or more activities. Interleukin 2 (IL_2) is produced by T cells activated by IL_1 and is responsible for T cell growth. B cell growth factor stimulates B cell growth. Macrophage migration inhibition factor, activating factor, and aggregating factor all are very similar and keep macrophages in the area of inflammation. Lymphotoxin produces cell death. Transfer factor transfers delayed hypersensitivity to a nonreactive host. It is specific for the antigen that caused its generation. Other lymphokine functions probably are associated with IL_1 or IL_2. Interferon is a cytokine produced by leukocytes (α interferon). IL_2 influences the production of γ interferon. Interferon is generated in response to viral infections and is released from the cell to cause adjacent cells to produce interferon and suppress the expression of viral RNA. Gamma interferon activates natural killer cells.

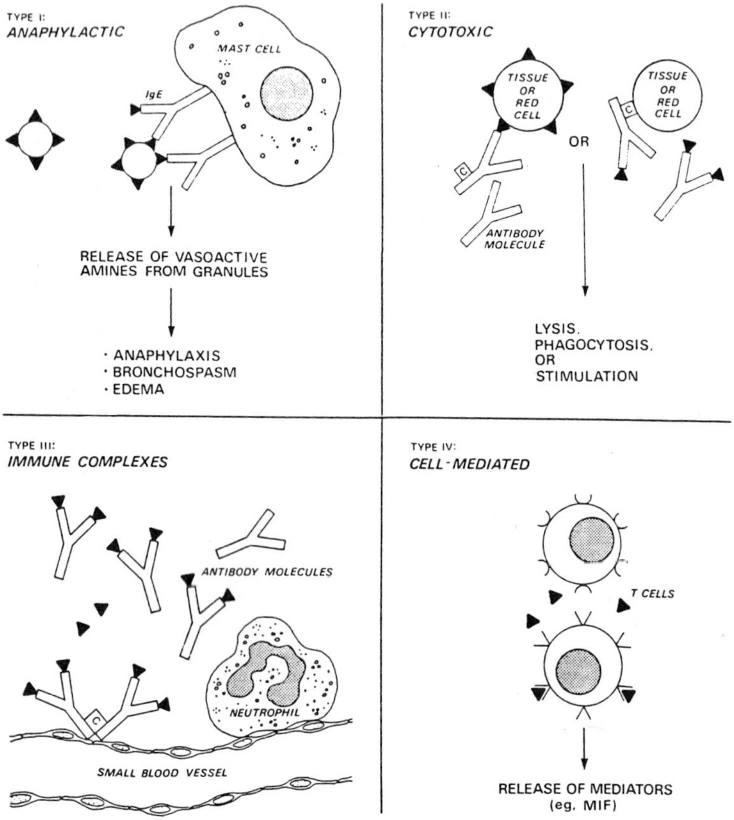

FIGURE 1–6. Schematic diagrams of the four types of immunologic mechanisms that may produce tissue damage. C = Complement; ▲ = antigen; U and V = specific receptors for antigens. (Reproduced with permission from Wells, J.V.: Immune mechanisms in tissue damage. *In* Fundenberg, H.H., Stites, D.P., Caldwell, J.L., and Wells, J.V. (eds): Basic and Clinical Immunology (ed 3). Copyright Lange Medical Publications, 1980, p 192.)

Natural Killer Cells

Natural killer cells (NK) are mononuclear cells of uncertain origin that can cause spontaneous cytotoxicity. Killing is antibody-independent and does not require prior sensitization. Typically, virally altered cells or tumor cells are affected. These cells are activated by γ interferon.

Killer Cells

Killer cells are lymphoid cells without the typical markers of B or T cells which have F_C receptors on the cell surface. These cells are responsible for antibody-dependent, cell-mediated cytotoxicity.

Immune Mechanisms Associated with Tissue Damage

The immune response is both protective and destructive. In beneficial immune responses, some local tissue damage occurs but it is minimal and easily repairable. In certain disorders, especially those associated with allergy or autoimmunity, the destructive effects predominate. Gell and Coombs classified these destructive responses into four types (Fig. 1–6).

Type I: Anaphylactic

Type I reactions are those of immediate humoral hypersensitivity associated with mast cells or basophil degranulation. Allergic disorders such as urticaria, atopy, and food hypersensitivity are examples of anaphylactic reactions.

Type II: Cytotoxic

Cytotoxic reactions are antibody-dependent; the antibody binds to cellular antigens or complement and causes cell death by phagocytosis following the activation of complement or killer cells. Examples of type II reactions include pemphigus and autoimmune hemolytic anemia.

Type III: Arthus (Immune-Complex)

Type III reactions are associated with soluble circulating immune complexes. These antigen-antibody complexes lodge in small blood vessels or in the glomerulus of the kidney where the basement membrane is not covered by cells. These trapped complexes activate complement, causing local vasoconstriction that favors further immune complex deposition. Additionally, complement activation attracts neutrophils that subsequently damage the tissues. Systemic lupus erythematosus is an example of a type III reaction.

Type IV: Cell-Mediated (Delayed)

Type IV reactions are cell-mediated; sensitized lymphocytes react with tissue-associated antigens and destroy them via the secretion of lymphokines or direct cellular effects. Allergic contact dermatitis is an example of a type IV reaction.

2 Urticaria, Angioedema, and Atopy

INTRODUCTION

Urticaria, angioedema, and atopy are type I hypersensitivity disorders in which the tissue reaction occurs within minutes after the antigen combines with its appropriate antibody. Mast cell or basophil degranulation is the central feature of anaphylactic hypersensitivity disorders. Anaphylactoid reactions are clinically indistinguishable from anaphylactic reactions but have no immunologic basis for the cellular degranulation. Anaphylactic reactions can occur focally, which is the basis of the allergy skin test, or in a generalized fashion. In animals, urticaria, angioedema, anaphylaxis, and atopy are pure type I hypersensitivity disorders. Food hypersensitivity and flea bite hypersensitivity may involve type I reactions, but other immunologic mechanisms may also occur so these are discussed separately.

PATHOMECHANISM

Immunologic mast cell degranulation is the initial pathologic event in anaphylactic reactions and is mediated by cytotropic reaginic antibodies. Although IgE is the classic reaginic antibody, other immunoglobulins may also be important, as is discussed later. Prior to mast cell degranulation, the patient must become sensitized to the allergen and form IgE antibodies.

All immunologically normal individuals can produce IgE antibodies but allergic patients have an exaggerated tendency to do so to normally innocuous substances. The scheme for the regulation of IgE production is shown in Figure 2–1. The allergen is processed by the macrophage, which then activates the T_H cell. This cell then activates the B cell to produce IgE. The T_S can interrupt this process by blocking the activation of the T_H cell, by interfering with the T_H and B cell interaction, or by directly inhibiting B cell differentiation. In humans, there is a tendency for allergic patients to have high serum IgE levels, while nonallergic individuals have low levels.

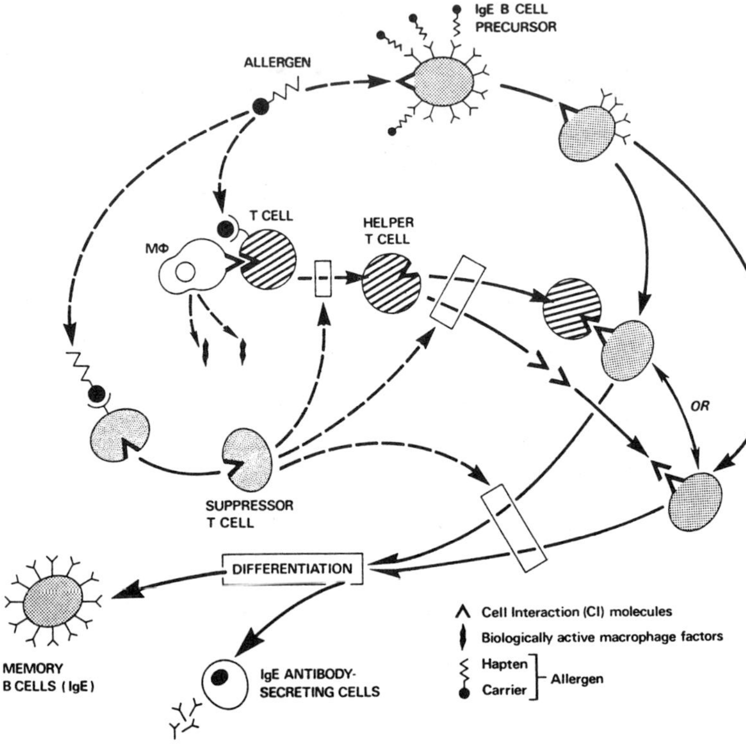

FIGURE 2–1. The IgE antibody-producing apparatus. (Reproduced with permission from Katz, D.H.: The immune system: An overview. *In* Fundenberg, H.H., Stites, D.P., Caldwell, J.L., and Wells, J.V. (eds): Basic and Clinical Immunology (ed 3). Copyright Lange Medical Publications, 1980, p 6.)

Since decreased allergen-specific T_S cell activity can be found in atopic patients, high levels of IgE would be expected. This control mechanism has not been studied in dogs.

In normal dogs, serum IgE levels vary from 30 to 350 μg/ml ($\bar{X}$ = 198). Vriesendorp found mean serum IgE levels of 198.8 μg/ml in normal dogs as compared with levels of 180.4 μg/ml in atopic dogs. Schwartzman studied the IgE levels in 70 dogs born to atopic parents and found mean levels of 125.4 μg/ml in affected dogs, 130.0 μg/ml in skin test–positive but clinically normal dogs, and 100.6 μg/ml in skin test–negative, clinically normal dogs. He also found that IgE levels decreased with age, which supports the finding of

Halliwell that the number of IgE-producing cells can decrease with age. Schwartzman also noted the tendency for IgE levels to increase with the duration of clinical signs.

The most probable explanation for why normal dogs have high IgE levels is the high incidence of external and/or gastrointestinal parasitism. In the atopic dog, parasite-induced elevations of IgE would mask rises caused by environmental allergens, and thus the measurement of total serum IgE is of little diagnostic significance. Measurement of antigen-specific IgE levels may be useful and is the basis for RAST and ELISA testing (see Ch. 4).

In the dog's skin, IgE binds only to mast cells. The binding of IgE to the cell surface receptors is reversible and, in humans, the affinity constant is so high that IgE tends to remain bound to the cell. Because of the high affinity constant, the half-life of IgE in human skin is from 8 to 14 days as compared with a serum half-life of 2.7 days. P-K testing in dogs supports a high affinity constant in this species as well.

IgE molecules bind to mast cells that have surface receptors for the F_C portion of the molecule. In humans, it has been estimated that between 100,000 and 500,000 molecules of IgE can bind to one cell. For optimum mediator release it appears that a threshold number of antigen-specific IgE molecules must be bound to a cell. In humans, the binding of at least 2500 molecules of antigen-specific IgE is thought to be necessary for optimum mediator release. No such data are available for the dog.

For mast cell degranulation to occur, bridging of IgE molecules is necessary. Accordingly, the allergen must be multivalent and have a stable antigenic configuration. Univalent allergens can bind to IgE molecules but will not cause mast cell activation. Following the cross-linking of IgE molecules, the mast cell is very rapidly activated to release preformed mediators and to synthesize new compounds. The exact nature of the signal caused by the bridging of IgE molecules is unknown but probably involves adenyl cyclase activation, augmentation of phospholipid metabolism, and phospholipid methylation.

In his work on canine atopy, Willemse identified a reagin that showed no identity with human IgE, was resistant to heat and chemical inactivation, and had P-K and passive cutaneous anaphylaxis (PCA) reactivity different from that seen with IgE. He identified this antibody as IgG_d. Subclasses of IgG are homocytotropic, but mast cells have fewer IgG receptors than they do IgE receptors. The affinity constant for the binding of IgG is very low so the antibody diffuses away fairly quickly. Sensitization persists for hours or days and not weeks as it does with IgE so the IgG molecules have been termed short-term sensitizing antibodies. Short-term sensitizing antibodies have been found in some human patients with allergic diseases, and Willemse found that 89 percent of his atopic dogs had specific IgG_d antibody titers against one or more allergens. Control dogs had no measurable IgG_d levels, while 55 percent of skin test–negative but clinically affected dogs had elevated titers. These data suggest that immunoglobulins other than IgE may be involved in canine atopy.

Other factors can affect the mast cell and make it more or less sensitive to immunologic stimulation. In 1968, Szentivanyi proposed the β-adrenergic theory of asthma, which stated that the common factor responsible for the hyperreactivity of the airways of asthmatics might be a β-adrenergic receptor blockade. The autonomic nervous system is responsible for the visceral control of the body and is composed of the parasympathetic and the sympathetic or adrenergic systems. Adrenergically affected tissues include mast cells, lymphocytes, and polymorphonuclear leukocytes, and they have α and β receptors on their cell surfaces. Although exceptions do occur, α receptors mediate cellular excitation while β receptors are inhibitory. These receptors work in concert with each other via a check and balance system. Decreased β reactivity or β blockade would cause a commensurate α hyperreactivity.

Cyclic nucleotides play a central role in cellular function. Reactions that increase the intracellular level of cAMP or decrease the intracellular level of cGMP will stabilize cells, while actions that cause the reverse will labilize cells. Typically, α receptors mediate decreases in cAMP while β-receptor stimulation causes an increase.

Szentivanyi's theory was based on the observation that his experimental asthmatic animals showed a hypersensitivity to histamine and other vasoactive substances and a reduced response to β-adrenergic catecholamines. Subsequently, many investigators demonstrated various degrees of α hyperreactivity or β hyporeactivity. Lymphocytes from asthmatics have decreased basal levels of cAMP and show a damped increase in cAMP with catecholamine stimulation. A decreased number of β receptors on the cell surface of leukocytes has been demonstrated in some asthmatics and autoantibodies to β_2 receptors also have been reported.

A group of basenji-greyhound crossbreed dogs has been studied because those dogs are naturally allergic or can be sensitized to *Ascaris* antigen. These dogs show both nonspecific and allergen-specific airway hyperreactivity typical of asthma. Additionally, these dogs suffer from atopic-like dermatitis, which flares after each allergen challenge and abates without treatment after antigen withdrawal. With antigen challenge, these dogs release histamine and slow-releasing substance of anaphylaxis (SRS-A) and show increased pulmonary resistance and decreased dynamic compliance. The pulmonary response to antigen challenge is potentiated by the administration of propranolol, which is a β-adrenergic antagonist. These dogs also show a blunted increase in intracellular cAMP when they are given isoproterenol, a β-adrenergic stimulant. All these facts indicate that the β-adrenergic response of these dogs is abnormal and that the β-adrenergic theory of Szentivanyi has some applicability to the atopic dog.

There is considerable evidence that the β-adrenergic theory does not explain all aspects of atopy in humans. A spectrum of autonomic abnormalities can be demonstrated that, no doubt, influences the allergic state. An altered autonomic state would not negate other trigger mechanisms but rather would serve to amplify the allergic response. For example, mediator release from mast cells is controlled by cAMP. Histamine released from the mast cell acts via H_2 cell surface receptors to increase cAMP. Increased cAMP levels cause the stabilization of the mast cell with inhibition of further mediator release. Alpha-adrenergic receptors mediate decreases in cAMP while β-adrenergic receptor stimulation causes increases. A β receptor blockade would cause a compensatory α stimulation that would dampen the rise in intracellular cAMP caused by the histamine feedback. Thus, mast cell degranulation would continue for a longer period of time, and the allergic reaction would be more intense.

After mast cell degranulation is triggered, the vasoactive substances, chemotactic factors, and enzymes are released, and the synthesis of reactive lipids (PAF, leukotrienes, and prostaglandins) proceeds. The vasoactive substances cause immediate vasodilation and vascular leakage which produce the clinical wheal. Depending on the sensitivity of the patient, the antigen load, and the persistence of the allergen, the reaction may be terminated or may continue. The vasodilation and increased vascular permeability cause local tissue edema, which flushes the vasoactive substances away from the site. Histamine and prostaglandin binding to the mast cell receptors stabilize the cell or adjacent cells and further inhibit mediator release. Eosinophils, attracted to the area by ECF-A, inactivate SRS-A, histamine, bradykinin, and PAF and further block tissue damage. In very sensitive patients or in those with a high, persistent antigen load, the humoral amplification system may be activated. Neutrophils attracted by ECF-A, PAF, NCF, and LTB_4 from mast cells and by the chemotactants from the amplification system can cause tissue damage and continue the inflammatory response.

In the early part of this century, there were reports that suggested that fatty acid supplementation could be beneficial in the treatment of atopic dermatitis in humans. More recent work proposes that a biochemical abnormality in fatty acid metabolism occurs in some atopic patients and may cause some of the clinical manifestations of this disorder. It is theorized that a defect in the function of the Δ-6-desaturase enzyme exists and results in the formation of more inflammatory eicosanoids. As some allergic dogs stop scratching with certain fatty acid supplements, this abnormality may also exist in dogs.

Schwartzman reported that atopic dogs showed some hypersensitivity to histamine, which would make these dogs more responsive to mast cell degranulation. Willemse introduced the term histamine reactive value (R_H) into veterinary allergy, which is defined as the sum of wheal diameters (mm) from intradermal injections of 0.05 ml of histamine at concentrations of 0.01, 0.1, and 1.0 percent. He defined a value of 49.0 ± 2.5 for normal dogs. Skin test–positive atopic dogs had a value of 51.5 ± 9.0, while skin test–negative atopic dogs had a value of 48.9 ± 6.1. These data do not support the theory of histamine hypersensitivity.

URTICARIA-ANGIOEDEMA-ANAPHYLAXIS

Immunologically mediated urticaria, angioedema, and anaphylaxis are all type I hypersensitivity disorders that can be thought of as the same disease with a variation in severity and target organ.

TABLE 2–1. Major Etiologic Categories of Urticaria and Angioedema

Drugs
Foods
Inhalant allergens
Infections
Insect and arthropod bites and stings
Penetrants and contactants
Internal diseases
Complement activation processes
Urticarial vasculitis
Genetic factors
Hereditary angioedema
Familial cold urticaria
Vibratory angioedema
Familial localized heat urticaria
Syndrome of urticaria, deafness, and amyloidosis
Erythropoietic protoporphyria
$C3_B$ inactivator deficiency
Physical factors
Dermatographism
Delayed pressure urticaria
Cold urticaria
Localized heat urticaria
Cholinergic urticaria
Cold-induced cholinergic urticaria
Solar urticaria
Aquagenic urticaria
Exercise-induced anaphylaxis
Psychogenic factors

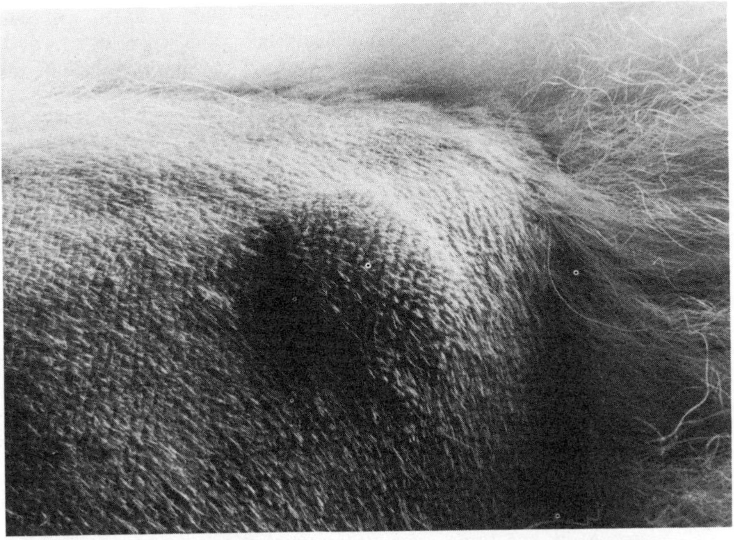

FIGURE 2–2. **A wheal caused by the intradermal injection of flea antigen in a hypersensitive patient.**

Nonimmunologic mechanisms also can cause these disorders; they are clinically indistinguishable from the allergic reactions.

Urticaria is a focal, superficial anaphylactic reaction that causes wheals (hives) to develop in the skin. Lesions may be singular or multiple and may affect the whole body. Angioedema reactions can be thought of as deep wheals. Deep blood vessels are affected, and the edema causes diffuse swelling usually in one area such as the head. Anaphylaxis is a severe systemic allergic reaction. In pets, the gastrointestinal tract is the "shock organ," and anaphylactic reactions cause contraction of the bowel smooth muscle and local vasodilation with splanchnic pooling of blood. As vasoactive substances are released into the circulation, generalized vasodilation can occur with hypotension and shock. Depending on the severity of the reaction, untreated anaphylaxis can be fatal.

These anaphylactic type reactions are uncommon in the dog and are rare in the cat. Ingestants (foods, ornamental plants, insects), drugs, vaccines, and venoms from stinging or biting insects are the most common causes. Factors important in humans are shown in Table 2–1. Reactions to inhalant allergens, allergy vaccines, infections, and physical stimuli have been recognized in pets. Type I hypersensitivity reactions occur within minutes after the antibody combines with the antigen. Injected allergens (drugs, vaccines, venoms) will cause reactions in the sensitized patient almost immediately. Ingested allergens (foods, drugs, and so forth) may not induce reactions for several hours and may persist for long periods until the allergen is completely absorbed or eliminated from the bowel.

Urticarial reactions (Fig. 2–2) are typically characterized by widespread, asymptomatic wheals which occur suddenly and will spontaneously regress as long as exposure to the allergen is eliminated. In long-haired animals, the reaction may not be observed. In short-haired pets, the lesions are more obvious (Fig. 2–3). The papular lesions of folliculitis sometimes are confused for urticaria. Urticarial lesions are usually not exudative and hairs cannot be easily epilated from them. Alternatively, folliculitis has both of these features.

Angioedema involves edematous swelling of a larger part of the body that also will spontaneously regress. An animal whose head or neck is involved (Fig. 2–4) should be watched carefully, as the respiratory tract may become obstructed via laryngeal tissue swelling. Anaphylactic reactions produce shock and are true medical emergencies.

For each of these disorders, the offending agent should be identified as subsequent exposures can produce more severe reactions. Mild reactions (asymptomatic urticaria, angioedema of a nonvital part of the body) require no treatment. Antihistamines will have no effect on pre-existing lesions but may prevent the development of new ones. Glucocorticoid steroids are beneficial. Serious

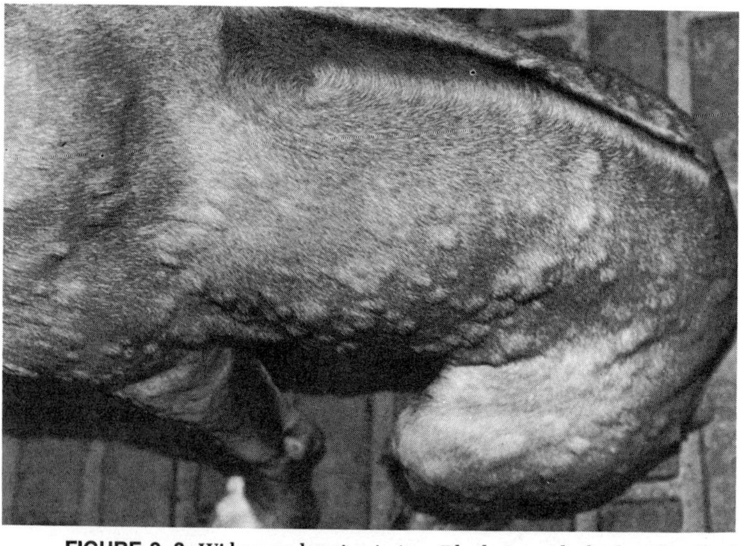

FIGURE 2–3. Widespread urticaria in a Rhodesian ridgeback with a food hypersensitivity.

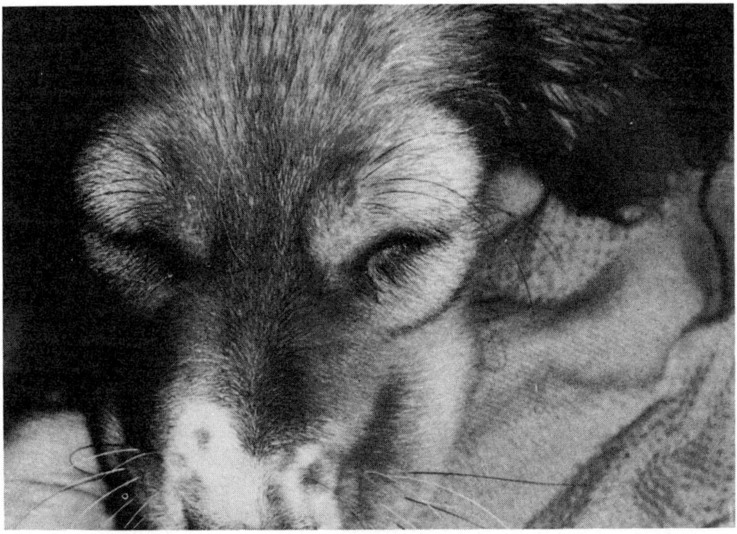

FIGURE 2–4. Facial angioedema due to an allergic reaction to a distemper-hepatitis vaccine.

reactions (anaphylaxis, angioedema of the larynx) require the use of epinephrine (1:1000) at a dose of 0.1 to 0.5 ml subcutaneously or intramuscularly, plus shock therapy if necessary. After the reaction is resolved, the offending agent should be avoided. If the animal is drug-sensitive, say to penicillin, that drug should be avoided and all similar drugs (semisynthetic penicillins and cephalosporins) should be avoided or used with caution since cross-reactivity could occur.

ATOPIC DISEASE

Atopy is a genetically determined predisposition to spontaneously develop type I hypersensitivities to normally innocuous substances. Offspring inherit the allergic predisposition from their parents, but siblings are not necessarily allergic to the same allergens. Genes confer the ability to hyperreact, while environmental exposure determines which allergens are significant. In humans, the term atopy is used to describe a triad of asthma, hay fever, and atopic dermatitis. In pets, atopy describes a pruritic dermatitis associated with the inhalation of pollen, fungal, or environmental allergens.

Canine atopy has been defined as an inherited predisposition to develop IgE antibodies to environmental allergens. The genetically controlled production of IgE and its binding to mast cells are considered fundamental to canine atopy. In a closing remark concerning the inability of his group to develop an inbred line of atopic dogs, Schwartzman stated that atopy in the dog may have multiple etiologies including nonallergic ones and/or that the trait cannot be inbred. Clinical and immunologic data support the concept of an inherited immunologically influenced disease, but the work of Schwartzman, Willemse, Hirshman, and others suggests that the IgE-mast cell theory may be too simplistic. As viral diseases or vaccinations can influence the cell-mediated immune system and, therefore, indirectly IgE production, environmental factors may also be important.

Since atopy is a newly recognized disease of the cat, our knowledge of feline atopy is much more limited. The inherited predisposition and the role of reaginic antibody remain to be proven.

HUMAN ATOPY

In the United States, it is estimated that between 10 and 20 percent of the human population suffers from some atopic disorder.

Asthma

Asthma is defined as recurrent episodes of wheezing or dyspnea characterized by a significant increase in airway resistance. Approximately 50 percent of the cases are believed to be caused by allergy, while the remainder are due to nonallergic, intrinsic, or infective factors. Allergic asthmatics show positive skin tests to the offending allergens and often have elevated eosinophil counts. The frequency and severity of asthma attacks may be greatly influenced by secondary factors such as temperature, humidity, exposure to noxious fumes, endocrine changes, and emotional stress.

Atopic Dermatitis

Human atopic dermatitis is a chronic inflammatory disease of the skin with certain characteristic clinical and morphologic features. Atopic dermatitis frequently occurs in patients with asthma or hay fever. Pruritus is a common presenting complaint. The atopic diathesis includes a cutaneous autonomic dysfunction and dry skin (xerosis) in which an itchy sensation can easily be provoked.

The precise etiology of atopic dermatitis is currently in doubt. Many investigators question the role of allergy in this disorder and believe it to be due to a genetically determined metabolic defect that alters the intrinsic itch threshold of the skin. The major argument against an allergic etiology is that there is poor correlation between symptoms and skin test or serologic allergy test results.

There is evidence for a depressed cell-mediated immune system in patients with atopic dermatitis and an increased susceptibility to cutaneous bacterial infections. Patients often have elevated IgE antibody levels to *Staphylococcus aureus,* and this organism can usually be isolated from affected skin. This also appears to be true in patients with allergic rhinitis.

Allergic Rhinitis (Hay Fever)

The term hay fever was based on the occurrence of a "strange disease" during the time of the year that coincided with the baling of grass hay. Many cases of hay fever as well as some cases of asthma are caused by inhalant allergies to nonpollens such as dust, molds, and animal danders. For this reason, the more specific term allergic rhinitis is preferred over hay fever or pollenosis.

Allergic rhinitis primarily affects the upper respiratory tract and may be seasonal or perennial. It is the most common of the human atopic disorders and affects approximately 15 percent of the United States population. There usually is good correlation between history, symptoms, allergy test results, and provocative exposure. These patients have a higher incidence of depressed cell-mediated immunity and have a lower resistance to minor infections.

CANINE ATOPY

Atopy is the second most common allergic skin disease of the dog. The true incidence of the disease in the dog population is unknown but estimates vary from 3 to 15 percent. A higher incidence of 30 percent has been reported for referral practices; this indicates the refractory nature of the condition. The disorder has been recognized worldwide.

Sociologic Data

Atopic disease can be recognized in dogs of any breed, but because of the genetic predisposition, the disorder occurs more frequently in certain breeds. Many reports fail to compare the incidence of the disease in a breed with the incidence in the general population, so the true breed incidence is difficult to assess. The reports by Halliwell and Scott indicate a breed predilection for the Boston terrier, Cairn terrier, dalmatian, English bulldog, English setter, Irish setter, Lhasa apso, miniature schnauzer, pug, Sealyham terrier, Scottish terrier, West Highland white terrier, and the wirehaired fox terrier. Both authors found a decreased incidence in the poodle, cocker spaniel, and dachshund. Halliwell recognized a low frequency in the German shepherd and Doberman pinscher, and Scott reported a low incidence in the German shorthair pointer. In 1983, Willemse reported a predisposition for the German shepherd, poodle, and boxer. In 1986, Schick added the golden retriever to the list of predisposed breeds but did not indicate an increased prevalence in the poodle, pug, German shepherd, cocker spaniel, bulldog, schnauzer, Doberman pinscher, mongrel breeds, and terriers other than the Cairn terrier and West Highland white terrier.

The apparent discrepancies in some of these reports can be explained by variations in breed popularity in a particular practice area, the breeding practices in that local area, or both. Limited breeding studies show that the progeny of atopic dogs are more likely to develop atopic signs, but the mode of inheritance is unknown. A relationship between dog leukocyte antigen (DL-A) typing and atopy was not found. If conscientious breeders of a certain breed of dog are aware of the inherited predisposition to atopic disease, careful breeding programs can decrease the incidence of the disease in a practice area. Alternately, poor breeding scruples can increase the incidence. Increased popularity of a specific breed is likely to increase the incidence of atopy because the population base increases and monetary considerations encourge the unrestricted breeding of unfit dogs. The increasing frequency of atopy in the Shar Pei exemplifies one of the detrimental effects of breed popularity or uniqueness. Both authors of this text are recognizing an increased frequency of atopic signs in the cocker spaniel and German shepherd.

Atopy can be recognized in dogs of any breed, even mongrel dogs. The authors have seen atopic signs spontaneously develop in multiple, unrelated dogs of different breeds within the same household. These findings suggest that factors other than genetics may be important.

Various studies have shown increased incidence of atopy in females while other studies refute these findings. Since estrogens can elevate intracellular cGMP levels and consequently labilize cells, an increased incidence in females would be plausible.

Age of Onset and Seasonality

The age of onset for atopic signs typically is reported to be between one and three years of age. Most studies report that approximately 75 percent of the atopic patients will show signs by three years of age. Willemse reported that approximately 27 percent of his patients developed their signs by one year of age, while Scott found that 64 percent of his patients developed their signs in this period. Vollset reported that he recognized atopy in a dog in which signs started at five months of age, and both authors have seen atopy in three-month-old dogs. After three years of age, the incidence of onset of atopy decreases, and the condition rarely starts in the dog older than six years.

Since sensitization is necessary before clinical hypersensitivity can occur, it is very unusual to see atopy in dogs younger than six months old. Approximately 78 percent of atopic dogs will first show signs during pollen seasons (spring to fall), so one would expect that the first pollen season (during the first year of life) would be used for sensitization. In highly inbred atopic dogs, the sensitization period may be weeks instead of months, so atopic disease can first appear early in life.

Van Stee made an interesting observation that a higher proportion of atopic dogs were born during the months of May, August, and December. This statistically significant increased incidence of atopy in dogs born during the onset of the major pollen seasons suggests that dogs may be particularly susceptible to primary sensitization during the first four months of life. Birth during nonpollen seasons would tend to disfavor the development of sensitization, while birth during pollen periods may increase the incidence of sensitization. This point would have impact on breeding programs. A preliminary study by one author (WHM) supports the observations of Van Stee.

It is rare to see atopic signs first develop in a dog after eight years of age. Unless a dog lives in a nonallergenic environment, signs should occur at an earlier age. Often careful examination of the history will indicate that the dog did show signs at an earlier age but that these signs were very mild. Allergic patients will often improve if they move to a different botanic area. This improvement usually will not be permanent as the patient most likely will become sensitized to the allergens in the new environment. Dogs who are moved frequently when they are young may not show significant clinical signs until they are older. True, sudden onset of atopic disease in an older dog that has been in the same environment all of its life probably reflects some change in or insult to its immune system. One author (WHM) reported one dog in which atopic signs did not become apparent until the dog developed pemphigus foliaceus.

Aeroallergens exist in the external and internal environment but there are many more pollens than there are household or indoor allergens. Accordingly, most atopic dogs would be expected to first show signs of disease during the warm weather. Scott reported that 78 percent of his atopic patients first exhibited signs of disease from spring to fall, while 22 percent developed signs during the winter. One would expect that most dogs with early atopy would show their signs seasonally. Scott reported that 42 percent of his patients exhibited seasonal pruritus but that 15 percent progressed to perennial disease. Thus at presentation to Scott 73 percent of the dogs were nonseasonally pruritic. This figure correlates well with the 72 to 76 percent incidence cited by Nesbitt and others. This high incidence of nonseasonal disease probably reflects the fact that mildly, seasonally pruritic dogs are not presented to veterinary dermatologists for skin testing. As the pruritic season expands or the animal's response to medical therapy decreases, the owners then seek specialized testing and therapy.

Threshold Theory

Each animal will tolerate some level of a pruritic stimulus without itching. If the stimulus exceeds the animal's threshold, itching will occur. The threshold for pruritus is very individualized and can be raised or lowered by psychologic changes as well as by physiologic alterations associated with nutrition, systemic disease, or environmental changes. Nervous or high-strung animals tend to itch sooner or more intensely than more placid dogs. A subclinical atopic pruritus may become clinical if the animal develops a secondary disorder such as seborrhea.

If an animal has only one type of allergy, e.g., atopy, the point at which the threshold is exceeded depends on the pollen load. A high pollen load will cause signs while a low load may be tolerated asymptomatically. A more interesting phenomenon occurs in animals with more than one form of allergy, e.g., atopy plus food hypersensitivity. If the intensity of each form of allergy is below the animal's threshold, the dog will not scratch, but if the two occur simultaneously, pruritus results. One author (WHM) has seen a ragweed-sensitive dog (skin test positive) that itched during ragweed season and that also had a food hypersensitivity. If the dog was fed a hypoallergenic diet during ragweed season, the atopic signs disappeared. Once ragweed season was over the dog could be returned to its original "allergic" diet without any sign of pruritus until the next ragweed season. Both authors have seen dogs in which atopic signs became evident only when the dog's flea bite hypersensitivity flared.

The threshold theory has diagnostic and therapeutic considerations. The clinical evaluation will suggest the diagnosis of allergy, but the clinician must decide if the animal has only one allergic disorder or more than one. In dogs with several different allergic conditions, elimination of one of the allergic disorders may cause the other allergic condition to become subclinical. If the second allergic condition does not become asymptomatic, the intensity of the pruritus should be decreased and the condition should be easier to manage.

The threshold theory also applies to animals with only one form of allergy. Successful immunotherapy to 10 allergens may eliminate the animal's pruritus even though the allergy test showed many more sensitivities. Elimination of the sensitivity to the allergens in the vaccine could decrease the pruritic stimulus to the point where it is below the animal's threshold.

Clinical Signs

The hallmark of atopy is pruritus that can be manifested by scratching, chewing, biting, licking, or rubbing. Some owners will deny a history of itching or pruritus until they are told that licking or rubbing is one of its signs. Some clients, especially first-time dog owners, do not recognize that some level of itching can be normal (physiologic pruritus). Physiologic pruritus is described as a sharp, well-defined pruritic sensation that is frequent but intermittent throughout the day. A normal dog can scratch occasionally, but it should be for brief periods of time and it should not interrupt normal activity. A dog who scratches frequently, focuses its attention on one spot, keeps the owner awake, or stops eating or playing to scratch has pathologic pruritus.

An occasional allergic dog will be presented with a history of pruritus of variable intensity but with absolutely no skin changes to support the complaint. Although the pruritus could be imagined by the owner, some dogs are poor scratchers and do not create lesions. Once one is sure that the owner understands the concept of physiologic pruritus, all cases of nonlesional pruritus should be evaluated for allergy before the complaint is dismissed as a psychologic problem of the owner or the dog.

Again, the primary sign of atopy is pruritus that initially is nonlesional. The dog starts to scratch at normal skin and lesions are caused by the dog. The classic atopic dog is described as one that scratches at its face, feet, and axillary regions, but a wide variety of signs can be recognized (Figs. 2–5 and 2–6). Most reports do not give a detailed description of the distribution of the lesions, so comparison is difficult. In his study of 100 atopic dogs, Scott reported that the initial pruritic sites were as follows: ventrum (35 percent); face, feet, and ventrum (22 percent); face and ventrum (12 percent); face and feet (10 percent); feet (10 percent); face (5 percent); feet and ventrum (3 percent); and ear (3 percent). As the disease becomes more chronic, the distribution becomes more widespread. Scott reported that, at presentation, 42 percent of the dogs had generalized pruritus, while the percentage of dogs who scratched at their face, feet, and ventrum increased from 22 to 31 percent.

Willemse's report on 208 dogs gives a detailed frequency distribution of the symptomatology, which is shown in Table 2–2. Although these data are not comparable with Scott's, similar trends can be seen. Facial and pedal pruritus was a consistent finding. He also noted frequent involvement of the extensor aspect of the carpal joints and the flexor aspect of the tarsal joints, which is a common finding in infantile atopic dermatitis in humans.

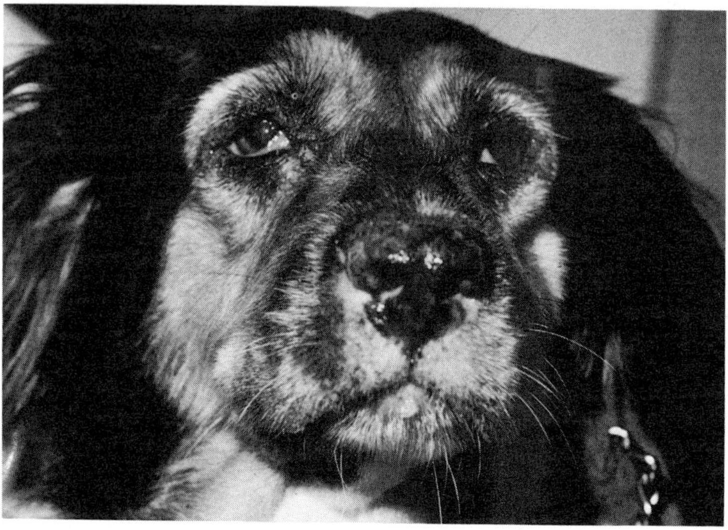

FIGURE 2–5. An atopic dog with periocular self-trauma, conjunctivitis, and rhinorrhea.

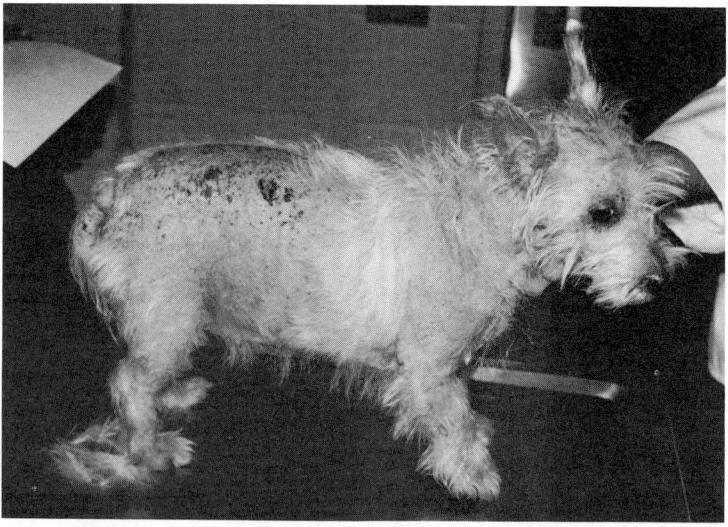

FIGURE 2–6. Generalized self-trauma in a chronically atopic dog.

TABLE 2–2. Frequency of Signs and Symptoms as Observed in 208 Dogs Having Atopic Dermatitis by Clinical Definition

Symptoms	Number of Dogs with Immediate Skin Test Reactivity (n = 170)	%	Number of Dogs without Immediate Skin Test Reactivity (n = 38)	%
Pruritus, face-rubbing, paw- and feet-licking	170	100.0	38	100.0
Bilateral conjunctivitis	51	30.0	11	28.9
Sweating	41	24.1	9	23.7
Sneezing	38	22.4	9	23.7
Discoloration of coat	13	7.6	3	7.9
Cutaneous involvement	161	94.7	37	97.4
Lichenification	143	84.1	33	86.8
Superficial pyoderma	45	26.5	4	10.5
Seborrhea	39	22.9	9	23.7
Affected skin regions				
Digits	124	72.9	28	73.7
Head	101	59.4	24	63.2
Extensor aspect, carpal joint	70	41.2	0	0
Axillaries	60	35.3	7	18.4
Flexor aspect, tarsal joint	52	30.6	0	0
Groins	31	18.2	7	18.4
Ear flaps	29	17.1	6	15.8
Abdomen	27	15.9	6	15.8
Flexor aspect, elbow joint	12	7.1	2	5.3

Reproduced with permission from Willemse, A., and Van den Brom, W.E.: Investigations of the symptomatology and the significance of immediate skin test reactivity in canine atopic dermatitis. Res Vet Sci 34:261–265, 1983.

While the majority of atopic dogs will show skin signs, some are presented only for otitis externa. Respiratory signs are uncommon and can occur with or without cutaneous signs. Typical respiratory signs, such as rhinitis or sneezing, involve the upper airway but an asthmatic dog occasionally can be identified. Dogs with respiratory signs only usually do not show significant skin test reactions. In humans, conjunctivitis can occur with the respiratory signs and mimic hay fever. The incidence of conjunctivitis in dogs is reported to vary from 30 to 50 percent.

Aside from skin and respiratory signs, canine atopy has been reported to be associated with a variety of noncutaneous disorders such as infertility, epilepsy, cataracts, gastrointestinal disease, and urinary tract disorders. If these disorders are of an allergic basis, their frequency appears to be low. It is more likely that these noncutaneous disorders are side effects of the medications used to treat the atopy.

History

A detailed history is the single most important factor in the diagnosis and management of an atopic case. It provides the key information to determine if the animal's symptoms have an allergic basis and, if so, what the most likely allergens are. If after the history and physical examination atopy is the most likely diagnosis, skin testing should be done. An accurate history is necessary to properly interpret the skin test results, as false-positive reactions can occur.

There is no ideal way to take an allergy history, but the owner's observations, the pet's medical record, and the veterinarian's own questioning all provide valuable information. Many clinicians ask the owner to fill out a history sheet before the animal is taken to an examination room. An example of such a form is shown in Table 2–3. Sometimes it is necessary to remove the pet from the owner so that he can concentrate on the history. If the animal is referred or has been treated by other veterinarians, the owner should be asked to bring a copy of the pet's medical record.

Once the client has provided the necessary information, the clinician should review it before the pet is examined so that confusing points can be clarified and additional information can be obtained during the examination. It is useful to list the owner's complaints and observations in chronologic order so patterns can be identified.

The nature and distribution of the signs, the seasonality of the problem, and the animal's response to medical therapy are important points to review with the owner. An important feature of atopy is that it is a progressive disease and the symptoms worsen yearly. The signs during the first year may have been so mild that the dog required no treatment and the owner may forget this episode. The

TABLE 2–3. Allergy History Questionnaire

Owner's Name: ______________________________ Date: ____________

Pet's Name: ______________ Breed: ____________ Age: ______ Sex: ______

Primary Complaint: ____

If itching (scratching, rubbing, chewing, biting, licking), where?

_____ Face _____ Feet _____ Armpits _____ Rear _____ Generalized

Respiratory (wheezing, sneezing, coughing)? ____________________________

Date or age *first* noticed: ______________________________________

Are symptoms worse: ___ Spring ___ Summer ___ Fall ___ Winter ___ Year Round

Are symptoms getting worse? ___ Yes ___ No ___________________________

What aggravates symptoms? ______________________________________

What helps symptoms? ____

Do any of the following occur? ___ Sores ___ Scabs ___ Scaling ___ Hair Loss

___ Odor ___ Redness ___ Watery Eyes ___ Ear Problems ___ Sweating

___ Hives ___ Convulsions ___ Drinks Excessive Water ___ Ravenous Appetite

___ Vomiting ___ Diarrhea ___ Weight Loss ___ Weight Gain

When did you last see a flea on your pet? __________________________

What do you normally feed your pet (type and brand)? __________________

Is your pet allergic to any food? ___ Yes ___ No Specify ________________

Allergic to drug or medication? ___ Yes ___ No Specify ________________

Do you have other pets? ___ Yes ___ No ___ Cats ___ Dogs ___ Birds _____ Other

Do you know of any relatives of this pet that have skin problems?

____

Does any human member of the household have skin problems? ___ Yes ___ No

Where does this pet sleep? _____________________________________

Other illnesses and dates: ______________________________________

Does bathing help or aggravate? _________________________________

Previous medications (brand): ______ Shampoos ______ Dips ______ Sprays

__________ Powders __________ Ointments __________ Tablets or Capsules

Last dose given ____________ Response ____________________________

Injection ____________ Date ____________ Response ________________

Previous veterinarian ____

Previous tests/skin scrapings ____________ Cultures __________________

Blood ____________ Other ______________________________________

Previous diagnosis: ____

What do you think is the cause of this problem? _____________________

owner should be questioned about earlier mild signs. Seasonal or perennial atopic dogs will usually show an intensification of their signs during certain periods, and these should be noted.

Glucocorticoids are usually so effective in the early stages of canine atopy that failure to improve with adequate steroid therapy makes the diagnosis of atopy less tenable. On the other hand, the converse is not true. Secondary pyodermas are common in atopic dogs, and these infected animals do not respond as well to steroid therapy. Owners of steroid-nonresponsive atopic dogs should be questioned carefully about the drug regimen used and the state of the dog's skin when the steroids were used. Since canine atopy is progressive, steroid responsiveness usually will decrease with time.

The owner should be questioned carefully about sudden flares in the animal's condition. Allergen levels can vary from day to day and, accordingly, the dog's level of pruritus can change. Usually the change in the intensity of the pruritus is gradual over a three- to seven-day period of time rather than sudden. Dogs that suddenly worsen probably have developed a secondary pyoderma and/or have picked up fleas or another parasite.

Some dogs suspected of atopy scratch less when they are hospitalized or boarded at a kennel. This decrease in pruritus could reflect the avoidance of a local allergen, poor observation, or an increase in the pet's allergic threshold via stress. Improvement in the patient's condition while it is away from home does not prove or disprove atopy.

Once the history and physical examination are completed, the clinician should have a good idea of whether the dog is allergic. Since it is not unusual for a dog to have two or more concurrent allergic conditions, it may only be possible to present the owner with an ordered list of differential diagnoses. When appropriate, allergy testing is done. After the results are available, more historical information will be necessary to see if the dog is exposed to the positive reactants.

Physical Findings

Primary lesions do not occur in atopy, or if they do, they may be masked by signs of self-trauma. The distribution of the lesions will be the same as the distribution of the pruritus. In mild cases, one may merely see broken hairs or salivary discoloration (rust-colored) of the fur. In more severe cases, one finds traumatic alopecia, erythema, and scaling of the involved skin. Chronically affected skin will be lichenified and hyperpigmented.

Secondary problems of seborrhea, pyoderma, or both are common in atopic dogs. These conditions themselves can be pruritic and they may lower the dog's allergic threshold. Hyperhidrosis (sweating) can be seen.

Special mention must be made of otitis externa, pododermatitis, acute moist dermatitis (hot spots), and acral pruritic nodules (lick granulomas). Otitis externa is a common finding in atopic dogs and can be the only sign of the disorder. Scott reported that 55 percent of his patients had otic disease and that it was the only clinical sign of atopy in 3 percent of the dogs. The ears are erythematous, waxy, edematous, and pruritic. Unless a secondary infection is superimposed on the allergic otitis, the condition is minimally exudative.

Resolution of any secondary infection will decrease the exudation but not the pruritus unless the otic preparation contains steroids.

Pedal pruritus also is common in atopy. Willemse reported that approximately 70 percent of his cases had pedal involvement. Scott also indicated a high incidence involving this site and noted that 5 percent of his cases had just pedal involvement. Pododermatitis or interdigital pyoderma can follow the pruritus, so atopy must be considered in dogs with infection of the feet.

Most atopic dogs traumatize regions of their bodies and do not focus their attention on just one spot. Dogs with true recurrent episodes of acute moist dermatitis can be suffering from atopic disease, food hypersensitivity, flea bite hypersensitivity, or a wide variety of other disorders and should be evaluated appropriately. The acral pruritic nodule is typically a focal area of disease on one or more limbs. Atopic dogs usually do not scratch at just one leg, but many scratch more intensely at one side of the body than the other. If the dog fixates on one spot, e.g., the extensor aspect of the carpal joint, an acral pruritic nodule may be created. However, the history or physical examination should indicate that the dog is more generally itchy and should be evaluated as allergic.

The physical trauma from scratching disrupts the integrity of the stratum corneum so atopic dogs are predisposed to secondary pyodermas and contact dermatitis. A drug or chemical, such as a medicated shampoo or insecticidal dip, may produce a dermatitis when applied to atopic skin. Any atopic dog whose condition worsens without an appropriate environmental reason should have its drug therapy—both topical and systemic—evaluated.

Differential Diagnosis

The list of differential diagnoses can be short or long depending on the physical findings. A list of common pruritic disorders of the dog is shown in Table 2–4. Dogs with nonlesional pruritus are candidates for atopic disease, food hypersensitivity, early flea bite hypersensitivity, intestinal parasite hypersensitivity, hormonal hypersensitivity, contact dermatitis, hookworm dermatitis, or *Pelodera* dermatitis. The reader is referred to the appropriate chapter for a complete description of the allergic disorders.

When lesions are present, the list of differential diagnoses expands to include sarcoptic mange, flea bite hypersensitivity, bacterial folliculitis with or without a hypersensitivity component, seborrhea, and the various immune-mediated disorders. The authors have examined many dogs suspected of having intractable atopic disease which actually have sarcoptic mange. Interestingly, some of these dogs were atopic but probably became infested at the grooming parlor, boarding kennel, or veterinarian's office. Sarcoptic mange

TABLE 2–4. Pruritic Disorders of the Dog

DISEASE	PRIMARY LESIONS PRESENT	LEVEL OF PRURITUS	RESPONSE OF PRURITUS TO STEROIDS	SITES OF PREDILECTION
Atopy	No	Mild to intense	Excellent	Face, ears, feet, axillae, anywhere
Flea bite hypersensitivity	Yes	Moderate to intense	Good to excellent	Lower back, thighs, ventrum
Food hypersensitivity	No	Moderate to intense	Variable	As in flea bite hypersensitivity or atopy, anywhere
Hormonal hypersensitivity	No	Intense	Poor	Lower back, perineum, ventrum
Contact dermatitis	No	Moderate	Poor to good	Feet, ventrum, perineum
Internal parasite hypersensitivity	No(?)	Moderate to intense	Poor to good	Flanks, lower back, perineum
Drug hypersensitivity	Yes	Variable	Poor	Anywhere
Psychogenic pruritis	No	Mild to intense	Poor	Feet, flank folds, perineum, tail
Sarcoptic mange	Yes	Intense	Poor	Ears, elbows, hocks, and ventrum
Cheyletiella dermatitis	Variable	None to intense	Good	Dorsum
Otodectic mange	No	Mild to moderate	Good to excellent	Ears, trunk
Demodicosis	Yes	Variable	Poor to good	Face, feet, anywhere
Pelodera dermatitis	No	Moderate to intense	Good	Feet, ventrum, perineum
Hookworm dermatitis	Yes	Moderate to intense	Poor to good	Feet, ventrum, perineum
Bacterial folliculitis	Yes	None to moderate	Poor to good	Anywhere
Bacterial hypersensitivity	Yes	Moderate to intense	Poor	Anywhere
Seborrhea complex	Variable	Mild to intense	Good	Face, ears, intertriginous areas, anywhere
Immune-mediated disorders	Yes	None to intense	Poor to good	Head, feet, ventrum, anywhere
Subcorneal pustular dermatosis	Yes	Mild to intense	Poor	Face, trunk
Cutaneous lymphomas	Variable	Moderate to intense	Poor to good	Face, anywhere

should be suspected in any severely affected "atopic" dog or in any true atopic that worsens suddenly.

Diagnosis

The diagnosis of atopy is based on the history, physical findings, elimination of the appropriate differential diagnoses, and allergy testing that correlates with the history. If allergy testing cannot be done, the other diagnostic steps should be taken to make the tentative diagnosis as firm as possible. Patients referred for allergy testing should be thoroughly evaluated for other allergic and non-allergic causes of pruritus before the referral.

Skin scrapings and fecal flotations should be done on all cases. Blood work usually is unrewarding, as eosinophilia is uncommon in dogs. In humans, some patients with an IgA deficiency have elevated IgE levels. If the atopic suspect gets disproportionally severe pyodermas, an immunoglobulin quantitation should be requested. Total serum IgE measurement is of little value as the levels in normal and atopic dogs often overlap. Skin biopsies show a superficial, perivascular dermatitis that is not specific for atopic disease but will support that diagnosis.

Dogs with pyoderma should be treated in an appropriate fashion to determine the significance of the infection. Atopic dogs frequently are secondarily infected, and the pyoderma intensifies and/or masks the signs of the atopic disease. Antibiotic therapy should lessen but not eliminate the pruritus in an atopic dog. If the pruritus is completely eliminated with the antibiotic therapy, the diagnosis of atopy is less likely. The authors have seen dogs in which the only sign of atopic disease was a recurrent generalized pruritic pyoderma. Although antibiotic therapy resolved both the pyoderma and the pruritus, the problem would recur. Skin testing showed significant reactions and immunotherapy resolved the problem. In these instances, the dogs were below their threshold level until the pyoderma appeared.

Since multiple forms of allergy can co-exist in a patient, all appropriate forms of allergy should be investigated. All dogs suspected of nonseasonal atopy should be checked for food allergy, even if they show positive skin test results.

As previously mentioned, the definitive diagnosis of atopy is made by allergy testing that correlates with the history. Although allergy testing usually will confirm the diagnosis, the real purpose for the testing is to start an immunotherapy protocol. If the situation is such that immunotherapy is inappropriate, there is very little value in conducting allergy tests.

FELINE ATOPY

There are ample clinicopathologic data to support the contention that atopy occurs in cats, but the genetic predisposition and the existence and role of reaginic antibody remain to be proven. In one study, Scott reported that 5 of 16 atopic cats had multiple relatives with a similar skin disorder. A reaginic antibody has been demonstrated in cats with ear mite hypersensitivity. This information suggests that the term atopy is applicable in the cat.

Clinical Features

Too few atopic cats have been recognized to make strong clinical statements. The age of onset is variable, ranging from 6 months to 8.5 years. Scott reported that 75 percent of his patients developed their clinical signs between 6 months and 2 years of age. No sex predilection has been mentioned.

The clinical presentation of an atopic cat is not as clear-cut as it is in the dog. Atopic cats can show lesional or nonlesional pruritus. Atopic signs include head and neck pruritus with or without rhinitis or conjunctivitis, miliary dermatitis, traumatic alopecia mimicking psychogenic alopecia, generalized pruritus, or lesions of the eosinophilic granuloma complex. If lesions of the eosinophilic granuloma complex are seen, they usually occur in conjunction with other skin lesions, especially those of miliary dermatitis. Much of the data presented on atopic cats deals with atopy-induced miliary dermatitis or psychogenic alopecia.

Atopic cats can exhibit their symptoms seasonally or perennially. Of the 16 cats studied by Scott with atopy-induced miliary dermatitis, 11 had seasonal signs (six warm weather, five cold weather), three had perennial signs, and two progressed from seasonal to nonseasonal. Since severely pruritic cats will mutilate their bodies, they are often presented to veterinary dermatologists early in the course of the disease so the true seasonality can be difficult to determine.

Response to steroids is a valuable clinical clue to the allergic nature of a cat's skin disease. Early on, atopic cats will respond well to corticosteroid administration, but as the disease becomes more chronic, the response can diminish. The authors prefer to use injectable methylprednisolone acetate (Depo-Medrol) at a dose of 5.5 mg/kg as the initial steroid. This dosage is very effective in the cat, and if the condition does not respond to it, then atopy is unlikely. Unfortunately, response to methylprednisolone does not mean that the cat is atopic but rather that it has a steroid-responsive condition.

Diagnosis

The diagnostic approach depends on the clinical presentation. Skin scrapings, fecal flotations, and fungal cultures should be run in all cases. Flea bite hypersensitivity should be evaluated by skin testing and/or trial flea control, and dietary allergy should be investigated by a dietary restriction. The next step depends on the clinical presentation and history. Cats with nonlesional pruritus or seasonal lesional pruritus should be skin tested. Cats with nonseasonal lesions of miliary dermatitis or the eosinophilic granuloma complex should be biopsied to eliminate the other causes of these disorders. Histopathology does not reliably distinguish between the miliary lesions of flea allergy, atopy, or food allergy. All cats with apparently idiopathic miliary dermatitis or chronic or recurrent eosinophilic ulcers, eosinophilic plaques, or linear granulomas should be skin tested.

3 Aeroallergens and Aerobiology

INTRODUCTION

Aeroallergens are airborne particles, such as pollens, house dust, mold spores, and animal danders, that are capable of eliciting an allergic reaction in a susceptible individual. Aeroallergens are complex particles that contain many molecular components, only some of which are allergenic. Most allergens have two or more antigenic determinants. Allergens typically are proteins or glycoproteins with a molecular weight of 20,000 to 40,000 daltons and vary in size from 2 to 60 microns. Larger particles have trouble reaching the terminal bronchioles and penetrating the mucous membranes. For a particle to be a significant aeroallergen, it must be antigenic, dispersible, and present in sufficient amounts.

AEROBIOLOGY

Aerobiology is the science of the origin, release, transport, and surface impact of windborne biological particles. Pollens and mold spores are typically studied, but other aeroallergens such as animal danders are also considered. Pollen or mold spore release is affected by wind, humidity, and temperature. Once a particle is airborne, it is subject to the effects of wind velocity, turbulence, rain, gravity, and atmospheric pressure. Dry, warm conditions with brisk winds favor pollen transfer, and pollens can travel several hundred miles. The pollen count in the vicinity of the plant is much higher and much more significant. Rainfall is thought to clean the air, but the cleansing effect depends on the duration of the rain and the droplet size. During thunderstorms, raindrops are usually large and will not remove much pollen. Prolonged rains often have smaller droplet size and can "scrub the air" effectively. Storms, whether they are brief or prolonged, can prevent pollens from reaching high altitudes and can concentrate the allergens lower to the ground.

Pollens and mold spores, identifiable by their microscopic appearance (Fig. 3–1), can be collected and counted by a variety of

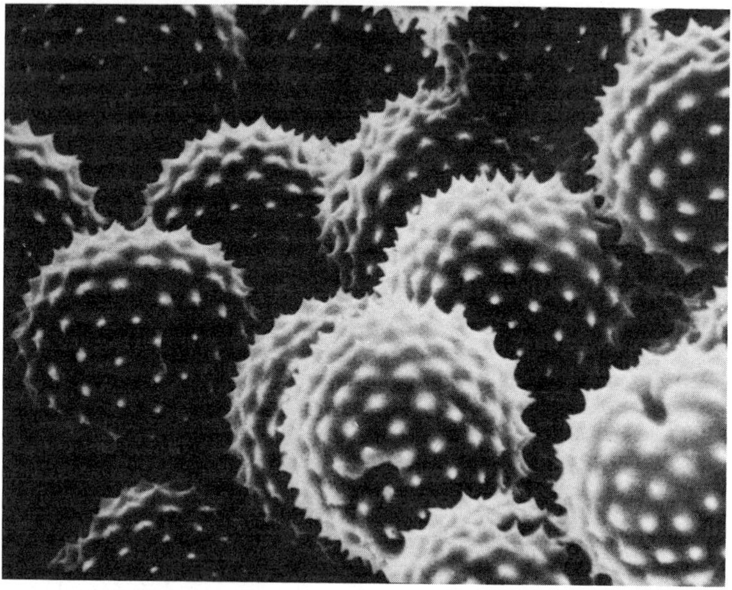

FIGURE 3–1. Scanning electron micrograph of ragweed pollen.

methods. So-called pollen counts are available from local weather bureaus. These data are most valuable in identifying which pollens and mold spores occur in a geographic area. If quantitative methods are used, the concentration of the various aeroallergens can also be determined.

Gravitational methods are the simplest but have many drawbacks. A slide coated with a soft glycerine jelly is exposed to the air for 24 hours; the pollens are identified by their morphology, and their numbers are counted. Slide placement is very important because wind velocity and direction greatly affect which pollens will be in the area. Since small particles are less affected by gravity, this method favors the collection of larger ones. Airflow is unknown, so pollen counts are unreliable. Volumetric methods involve the use of machinery that samples the air in known volumes. Smaller pollens will be collected with these methods, and pollen counts tend to be more reliable.

Pollen counts are most helpful in determining which pollens are in a geographic area. When pollen counts are low, many allergic patients will experience less intense symptoms, but symptomatology is not directly related to pollen count. Individual sensitivity combined with the local concentration of pollens is very important. Most pollens never reach the air but fall to the ground near the plant. Since dogs and cats are low to the ground and constantly sniff, they are exposed to many more pollens than humans.

POLLEN AEROALLERGENS

Pollen grains are essential for the reproduction of seed plants. Pollen transfer is accomplished by insects (entomophilous pollination), the wind (anemophilous pollination), or a combination of both. Entomophilous pollination typically occurs in plants that produce single, showy, colorful, and fragrant flowers. These plants have local allergenic potential for people or animals in their immediate vicinity but are insignificant away from the plant, since their pollens are large and heavy, have an adhesive coating, and are produced in small amounts. Anemophilous plants are usually drab, with many small, inconspicuous, and odorless flowers. Because of the relative inefficiency of wind pollination, these plants can liberate millions of pollen grains.

Pollen levels depend on the number of plants in an area and the efficiency of pollen release. Although some plants forcibly eject their pollens, most just drop the pollen. Pollens can fall onto leaves or to the ground. Pollens caught in vegetation are subject to wind dispersal, while pollen on the ground is lost. Dogs or cats who wander through fields are exposed to massive pollen loads from the ground.

For a pollen to be a major allergen, it should be allergenic, windborne, buoyant, and produced in large quantities by abundant, widely distributed plants. Ragweed is the best known example of a pollen that meets all these criteria. In humans, dandelion is not important since, although it is allergenic and abundant, it is rarely airborne.

Pollen shedding is not uniform throughout the day because it is affected by air temperature, humidity, and wind velocity. Rapidly moving air of low humidity promotes pollination. Typically, the best conditions for pollination occur at mid-day and in the afternoon when the air is warm and dry. Many plants have mechanisms to prevent pollen release when the humidity is high. Short ragweed pollen release is affected by diminishing day length, overnight rainfall, and temperature. As the overnight temperature rises and the humidity decreases, pollen release is triggered 1 to 3 hours after sunrise. Airborne levels increase 2 to 4 hours later as pollens on plant leaves dry out and become windborne. Because of their buoyancy, airborne pollens can travel for hundreds of miles. Ragweed pollens have been detected at altitudes of 17,000 feet and as far as 400 miles from land. Again, local concentrations are much more important.

Plant growth obviously affects plant pollination. Dry, cool weather limits plant growth; warm, wet conditions encourage it. Within any one of the botanical zones of the United States, there are certain growing seasons for the various plants. As a general rule, trees pollinate first in the spring, followed by grasses and then weeds. Molds, depending on their method of spore release, tend to peak during wet conditions in the spring and fall. During the early growing season, pollen production is scant. Pollen levels peak during the middle of the growing season and then gradually decrease. Although pollen grains are reproductively viable for only a few hours, their allergenicity lasts much longer. Frost will terminate pollination by killing the plant, but pollens already released will linger on dead plants and on the ground. In warmer climates, some plants will continue to pollinate year-round, although pollen levels will vary with the season and with local weather conditions.

The botanic classification of plants can be helpful in determining the allergenic potential of a plant. Plants are described by their order, family, genus, and species. For some plants, subspecies or varieties also exist. In large families, related genera may be grouped as tribes. Closely related plants may share some common antigens and may be cross-reactive.

Grasses

There are approximately 400 genera of grasses, all belonging to the same family, with at least 4500 species of anemophilous plants. Cultivated species are most important, and, worldwide, grass allergies are the most significant in humans.

Throughout the northeastern two-thirds of the United States and southern Canada, the bulk of windborne grass pollen is derived from bluegrass (Canada and June or Kentucky), orchard grass, timothy grass, and red top grass. The rye grasses, Italian or perennial, are also important. Bermuda grass is a major pollen source throughout the southern half of the United States and along the Pacific coast.

Most temperate zone grasses, except Bermuda grass, have some allergenic cross-reactivity. Grass pollen typically contains at least two antigens. One is specific for the individual pollen, while the other is common to the entire family. Rye grass has four group antigens, but one is nonallergenic or weakly allergenic. Rye Group I antigen, or one very similar to it, is found in most if not all grasses, except Bermuda grass. Group II antigen is prominent in rye, fescue, orchard, and velvet grasses, while timothy and sweet vernal are relatively deficient.

In the temperate regions of the United States, the peak pollen period for grasses is from mid-May to mid-July.

Weeds

Weeds are small annual plants that grow wild and have little or no agricultural or decorative value. The most important allergic group is the Compositae family, which includes 20,000 or more species and is divided into 14 tribes. The ragweed tribe (*Ambrosia*) is most important, and in the United States, ragweed is the major cause of hayfever in humans.

More than a dozen ragweed species are found in North America, but six are of major significance. Short, giant, slender, Western, Southern, and false (bur) ragweeds are widely distributed in the United States and adjacent Canada. Short and giant ragweed are the most prolific sources of pollen. Ragweed pollen contains approximately 14 soluble proteins and polypeptide antigens, but they are not all significant allergens. For short ragweed, at least five separate allergens have been identified. These allergens vary in their molecular weight, physical and chemical characteristics, speed of extractability, and heat lability. Certain patients will react to some antigens while others will not. The bulk of the allergenic activity is believed to be associated with a simple globular protein called Antigen E. Antigen E is 200 times more active than whole ragweed extract.

The pollens of the *Iva* species are similar in appearance and allergenic activity to ragweed. Rough marsh elder, burweed marsh elder (prairie ragweed), and povertyweed may cross-react in ragweed-sensitive patients. The same may be true for cockleburs.

The tansy tribe includes the sages, sagebrushes, wormwoods, and mugworts. Members of the dandelion tribe include dandelions, asters, goldenrod, sneezeweed, and dog fennel. Cultivated members include chrysanthemums, dahlias, and marigolds. These weeds and flowers typically are insect-pollinated and are not of major windborne significance except in the vicinity of the plant. Ragweed-sensitive patients may show a sensitivity to members of the dandelion tribe.

The goosefoot (Chenopodiaceae) family includes Russian thistle, burning bush (Kochia), salt bushes, smotherweeds, greasewood, lamb's quarter, and Mexican tea. The amaranth (Amaranthaceae) family includes pigweed and western waterhemp. These families produce similar pollens, and some investigations suggest strong interfamilial as well as intrafamilial similarities in their allergens. Sorrels and docks belong to the Polygonaceae family and seem to cross-react.

Over 90 weed and garden plant pollen extracts are available, and the nature of the allergens of these flowers is not well-defined. Ragweed Antigen E activity has been found in the various ragweed species, marsh elders, and cocklebururs, so these pollens may cross-react. Plants within the same tribe may also cross-react.

Trees

In general, the period of pollination of deciduous trees is brief and occurs shortly before, during, and shortly after leaf development. In more temperate climates, tree pollination is concluded by late spring. In warmer areas, this season may be extended. In some areas, conifers, especially mountain cedar, pollinate in the winter. As compared to weeds and grasses, tree pollens are less significant.

Two classes of trees, the Gymnospermae and the Angiospermae, are of allergenic significance. The Gymnospermae include the conifers, which produce vast amounts of pollens. Essentially, two major types of pollens are released by this class. Pines, spruces, firs, true cedars, black hemlock, and golden larch release large (50 to 90 microns), coarse-surfaced grains. Members of the cypress-juniper family, yew family, and the bald cypress-sequoia family share spherical pollen grains, 20 to 35 microns in diameter. Conifers that produce large pollens are of uncertain but probably limited allergenic significance to humans. The families that produce the smaller pollens tend to be more important. Mountain cedar, red cedar, ornamental yews, and junipers are examples of important conifers.

The Angiospermae are the conventionally flowering trees with many families and species. The Salicaceae family includes two genera: the willows *(Salix)* and the poplars and aspens *(Populus)*. The pollens of the two genera are dissimilar morphologically and probably in allergenic content as well. The *Populus* genus includes the poplars, aspens, and cottonwoods.

The Juglandaceae family includes the *Carya* and *Juglans* genera. The *Carya* genus includes the hickories and pecans, while the *Juglans* genus includes the walnuts and butternuts. The Betulaceae family includes the hazelnut and filbert *(Corylus)*, the birches *(Betula)*, and the alders *(Alnus)*. The Fagaceae family includes the oaks *(Quercus)*, the beeches *(Fagus)*, and chestnuts *(Castanea)*. Oak pollens are morphologically very similar. The Ulmaceae family includes the elms *(Ulmus)* and hackberries *(Celtis)*. The Oleaceae family includes the ashes *(Fraxinus)* and the olive tree *(Olea)*. The Aceraceae family includes maples and box elders. Insect pollination occurs with varying degrees in this family. The mulberry family (Moraceae) includes the mulberries *(Morus* and *Broussonetia)*, hemp *(Cannabis)*, hops *(Humulus)*, and Osage orange *(Maclura)*.

Presently, each tree pollen is thought to be antigenically different. If tree mixtures are to be used for testing or immunotherapy, species from one family should be grouped together.

Fungi

Fungi are universal in distribution, and fungal spores can comprise the bulk of the suspended allergenic particles in an area depending on the weather conditions and land usage. Most fungi of allergic significance are nonpathogenic saprophytes. Fungi reproduce by sexual and/or asexual methods. Many of the common allergenic fungi reproduce asexually. All fungi require oxygen for growth and grow best under warm and humid conditions. The majority of fungi become dormant at subfreezing temperatures but can survive prolonged freezing. Atmospheric moisture affects not only fungal growth and sporulation but also spore dispersal. Although the general atmospheric humidity may be very low, fungi may find free water for growth and sporulation in damp areas and thus can be found almost anywhere.

Some fungi shoot their spores into the environment, and this process requires free water. High levels of these spores occur with rainfall or fog or during the hours of darkness when humidity tends to increase. Levels of *Fusarium, Phoma,* and *Cephalosporium* peak with precipitation. Most fungi of allergenic significance disperse their spores in dry conditions. Spore dispersal increases as airspeed increases and humidity decreases. Maximum levels occur during sunny afternoon periods. Species of *Cladosporium* (formerly *Hormodendrum*), *Alternaria, Aspergillus, Epicoccum, Helminthosporium, Penicillium,* and *Rhizopus* use dry spore dispersal. Once a spore is airborne, it is subject to the same atmospheric effects as pollens.

Fungi are common indoors and outdoors. Some species are primarily field molds, while others will grow both inside and outside. Accordingly, symptomatology can be seasonal or perennial. Seasonal symptoms tend to peak in mid-summer and persist until well after a killing frost. Perennial symptoms can occur because most houses, especially those that are damp, have fungi growing in them. *Penicillium, Aspergillus,* and *Rhizopus* are common indoor "mildew" isolates. The following discussion highlights the important features of some fungi.

Alternaria grows on organic debris in the soil and parasitizes the leaves, stems, flowers, and fruits of many vegetables, cereal grains, and ornamental plants. The spores are common in the air from late spring to fall, especially from noon until 3:00 P.M. In humans, *Alternaria* is considered the most clinically reactive airborne fungus. *Aspergillus* is a common soil fungus that also grows in stored foods and on wet surfaces indoors (bathrooms, basements, and drip pans of refrigerators). *Aureobasidium (Pullularia)* is a soil saprophyte that grows on decaying vegetation. Spores peak in the afternoon. This fungus grows on caulking compounds, so it can be found in bathrooms. It also is found on paper, lumber, and paints. *Cladosporium* grows on organic debris in the soil and on dead leaves but also can be found on leather, rubber, cloth, paper, and wood products. This type of spore is very common in the air with peak levels seen from mid-summer through December. Peak daily levels occur between 11:00 A.M. and 3:00 P.M. *Curvularia* is a common parasite of grasses, and spores are dispersed by lawnmowing activities. *Epicoccum* is widespread in temperate regions, especially in grasslands and agricultural areas. It colonizes decaying vegetable matter, plant leaves, uncooked fruit, and textiles. Peak levels occur in late summer and in the fall. *Fusarium* species are parasitic on vegetable and field crops, and the fungus can be found on stored fruits and vegetables like cucumbers, tomatoes, and potatoes. Spore dispersal requires rain; therefore spores are common in the air after rainfall.

Helminthosporium is a prevalent outdoor fungus of grasses and cereal grains. Grain threshing releases large quantities of these spores. Natural spore release peaks around 2:00 P.M. *Mucor* is a soil saprophyte especially of leaf litter and organic debris and can be found on animal wastes. Spore levels in the air tend to be low. *Penicillium* is a fungus of the soil, fruits, breads, cheeses, and other foods. Airborne levels outdoors are low but are plentiful indoors during the winter. Patients allergic to this mold do not necessarily have an increased sensitivity to penicillin drugs. *Phoma* is found on certain green plants and on paper products such as books and magazines. *Rhizopus* is a common saprophyte of organic soil debris outdoors and can be found on cured meats, root vegetables, and bakery goods indoors. *Stemphylium* parasitizes leaves and stems of vegetable crops and also can be found in decaying plant material, damp paper, canvas, and cotton fabric. Its skin test cross-reactivity with *Alternaria* has been noted. These spores are fewer in number than those of *Alternaria* and are found during the daytime in the summer months.

Many more fungi exist than are listed above and may be of allergenic significance. Fungi contain weak antigens that, with rare exception, do not appear to cross-react. Mold allergens are prepared by different methods; those made from the powdered spore material are antigenically more active than those from the mycelium. One batch of a mold allergen can vary significantly from the next batch. These factors have made it difficult to determine the true incidence and significance of mold sensitivity in pets.

ENVIRONMENTAL ALLERGENS

This group of allergens includes dusts, danders, feathers, furniture stuffings, and a variety of other allergens. These allergens are usually associated with indoor symptoms. Depending on the animal's sensitivity, the signs can be seasonal or perennial. Although indoor allergens are present year-round, their relative concentrations are lower during the spring and summer months because houses are more open. As winter approaches, windows and doors are closed and concentrations start to increase.

House Dust

House dust is an important aeroallergen that is actually a heterogenous, ill-defined substance. House dust contains animal danders, molds, insect debris, bacteria, fibrous material of plant and animal origin, food remnants, and many other substances. Dusts from different parts of the world have a similar antigenicity. House dust extracts tend to be irritating and must be used carefully to avoid false-positive reactions. In humans, there appears to be some uniqueness to house dust antigen, which cannot be explained by its various ill-defined constituents.

House dust mites (arachnids) appear to be an important allergenic component of house dust. These mites live on epidermal debris from people and animals, yeasts, molds, and remnants of household foods. There are more than 36 species of mites in dust, but *Dermatophagoides farinae* and *Dermatophagoides pteronyssimus* (Fig. 3–2) appear to be most important. Mite reproduction is thought to be regulated by temperature and humidity; other factors are probably involved as well. The optimum conditions to culture *D. pteronyssimus* in the laboratory are a relative humidity of 50 percent and a temperature of 25° C. More mites are found on the surfaces of mattresses than on the floor, since epidermal cells are concentrated on mattresses. Mites are also more often found in damp (humid) houses than in dry ones. Thus, mite counts can vary with the local environmental conditions and with the source of collection. Mite allergenicity does not depend on the viability of the mite, as mite excreta and dead mites also are allergenic. The vigor of household cleaning and extermination does not appear to affect mite recovery rates.

The allergenicity of house dust increases when it is stored for several months before it is extracted. Inoculation of sterile dust samples with live house dust mites increases the skin test reactivity of the extract, and the increase in reactivity parallels the numbers of mites in the preparation. Most human patients who react to dust antigen also react to mite antigen but at much lower concentrations. Reactivity to dust mites has been reported in veterinary medicine, but the rate is lower than in humans. In animals and humans, dust mites are a major but not the only source of house dust allergen.

Other dusts such as barn and wood dust may be important depending on the animal's exposure. Other mites also can be significantly allergenic. Vollset reported on dogs that were allergic to storage mites found in poorly dried cereals.

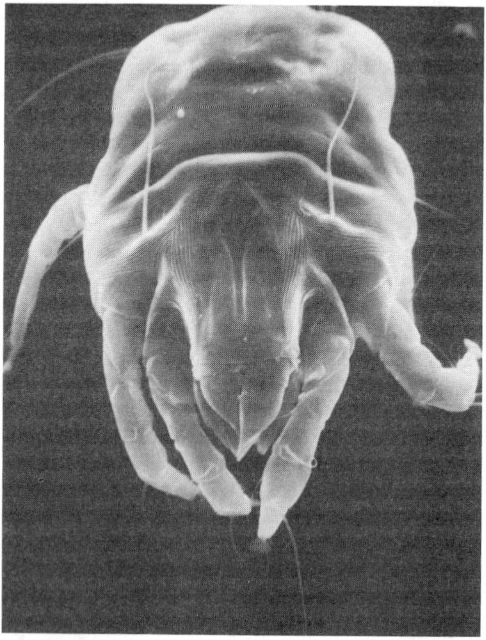

FIGURE 3–2. Scanning electron micrograph of *Dermatophagoides pteronyssimus*. (Photo courtesy of T.A.E. Platts-Mills, University of Virginia, Charlottesville, Virginia.)

EPIDERMAL ALLERGENS

Animals and humans constantly shed hair and dead epidermal cells into the environment. Hair is considered a minor allergen because it is less soluble and less airborne. Epidermal cells, or danders, are proteins with multiple antigenic determinants and often are contaminated with saliva, serum, or urine, which can increase the antigenicity of the dander. It has been shown that dander extracts vary depending on the method of extraction and also that there probably are allergens specific to one breed of animal. A person sensitive to dog dander can be more sensitive to one breed of dog than another, independent of the dog's hair length or shedding pattern. This phenomenon is suspected but not proved in other species of animals.

Cat Allergen

For humans, cats are more allergenic than dogs. Immunochemical studies have shown that the major allergen from cat pelts is cat allergen 1. This allergen is more potent than pure epidermal extracts and differs from serum proteins. The allergen is highly concentrated in the salivary glands. Allergens also are present in the urine and in the serum proteins. The grooming habits of the cat cause it to spread these allergens over its body and therefore increase its allergenicity. Drugs such as atropine, which decrease salivary secretions, inhibit the spreading of the antigen.

Dog Allergen

None of the allergens in dog dander has been isolated in pure form, but the allergenicity appears to be related to epidermal proteins plus several serum proteins. Breed variations in antigenicity do occur. The significance of a strong reaction to dog dander in a dog is uncertain.

Human Allergen

One person typically produces 5 grams of dander per week, so animals are exposed to high levels of this allergen. Surveys from veterinarians indicate frequent reactions to human dander. Presently extracts of human hair or dander are not marketed.

Other Epidermal Allergens

Extracts from the camel, cow, deer, fox, gerbil, goat, guinea pig, hamster, horse, mink, monkey, mouse, pig, rabbit, rat, and seal are available commercially. These allergens probably include not only epidermal antigens but also serum, salivary, or urinary antigens. A major allergen is found in mouse urine. Some human patients allergic to horses react to epidermal antigens as well as to serum proteins. In addition, patients who become sensitive to an animal dander may develop sensitivities to other products from these animals such as meat or antisera.

Since the use of horse and cattle hair as furniture stuffing or carpet matting is on the decline, the incidence of reactivity should also decrease. Pets in rural environments can be exposed to farm animals and can develop sensitivities to them.

Sheep's Wool

The true allergenicity of sheep's wool is debatable since wool is an irritating substance and extracts can contain not only wool but also dusts and danders from humans and other animals. Although skin test reactivity to wool is common in the dog, the significance of wool as an aeroallergen is uncertain.

Feather Allergens

Exposure to feathers in pillows, comforters, jackets, and quilts or by handling birds is known to cause respiratory and cutaneous allergic disease. Aged feathers are more allergenic than fresh-plucked feathers. Since antigenicity increases with age and many human patients show a strong correlation between skin test reactivity to feathers and house dust, it is theorized that house dust mites are responsible for the allergenicity of feather extracts. Work in patients with feather-induced hypersensitivity pneumonitis and chemical extraction studies show that feather extracts differ from house dust extracts.

Since feather allergen is believed to be a degradation product, most feather-allergic patients can eat fowl without fear of allergic cross-reactivity. Most commercial feather extracts are mixtures of chicken, goose, and duck feathers, since these feathers are commonly used for stuffings. The degree of antigenic cross-reactivity between these feathers and those from pet and wild birds is unknown. The authors have recognized cases of dogs that were allergic to the household parrot (proven by isolation) and that also reacted to mixed feather extract.

Kapok

Kapok is the moisture-resistant seed hair from the kapok tree which is used as a stuffing for furniture, mattresses, and aquatic life jackets or cushions. The use of synthetic fibers has markedly decreased the demand for kapok. As was true with house dust and feathers, the allergenicity of kapok increases with age because of house dust mite contamination and biologic deterioration.

Cottonseed and Flaxseed

The water-soluble, proteinaceous material from cottonseeds can contaminate inexpensive cotton stuffing and cause allergic signs. The use of synthetic fibers has decreased the incidence of reactivity to cottonseed.

Pyrethrum

Pyrethrums are widely used botanic insecticides produced from the flower heads of the Chrysanthemum cinerarie-folium plant. These plants are members of the Compositae family and are related botanically to ragweed. Patients allergic to ragweed may also be reactive to pyrethrum insecticides. Clinical allergy to these insecticides appears to be very low.

Tobacco

Tobacco smoke can be irritating, and it will cause many pets to sneeze. Inhalant allergies to tobacco smoke are rare but do occur. Because Scott reported a high incidence of false-positive reactions to tobacco, skin test results must be evaluated critically. One author (WHM) has seen two dogs that were apparently allergic to marijuana smoke.

INSECT ALLERGENS

Insect hypersensitivity typically is due to the bite or sting of the insect rather than the inhalation of insect-associated allergens. In humans, especially urban dwellers, cockroach antigen appears to be a significant allergen, and it is different from house dust antigen. Inhalation of insect debris from the caddis fly and mayfly also causes allergic symptoms.

Nesbitt reported a 60 percent reactivity to cockroach antigen in urban dogs. In rural New York, one author (WHM) has seen only one dog react to this antigen. The work of Nesbitt and Vollset, who studied storage mite hypersensitivity, indicates that inhalant insect hypersensitivity may be important in pets.

OTHER ALLERGENS

Various gums, glues, and fibers are available for allergy testing. The commercial availability of these products suggests that they are of potential allergic significance in pets. If the animal's exposure history indicates that one of these allergens may be important, the animal should be tested for it.

ALLERGEN PREPARATION

Simply stated, allergy extracts are prepared by collecting the material, extracting the "allergens," and mixing them with preservatives. The collecting and manufacturing techniques can vary among laboratories. Additionally, the allergenicity of one batch of an allergen can be significantly different from the next batch, even if it was produced by the same company. This variability reflects our ignorance of what the major antigenic determinants are in the various allergens and the biologic variability of pollens. Until all antigens are completely defined, all allergens should be purchased from the same allergy laboratory to maintain as much consistency as possible.

Pollen extracts are prepared by collecting the pollen, cleaning it if possible, and then drying it to prevent bacterial or fungal contamination. Prior to extraction, pollens often are defatted with various ethers and techniques. Careless defatting can remove some of the potential allergens. Fungal antigens are usually made from dried ground powders of the mycelial mat, but sometimes only the growth medium or the mat plus the growth medium is used. Allergens are extracted from the crude materials by the use of saline solutions to which other agents can be added. Once the extraction is completed, the allergen can be freeze-dried or diluted to the necessary strength. Sterility checks are run on each batch and after vialing.

To inhibit microbial contamination, preservatives are added to the extracts. Commercially, either 0.4 percent phenol or 50 percent glycerin is used. Some laboratories offer extracts preserved with 0.03 percent human serum albumin, but these have not been investigated in animals. Preservatives not only inhibit microbial growth but also affect the stability of the extracts.

STABILITY OF ALLERGENIC EXTRACTS

Allergy extracts are dated biologic materials that will start to lose potency within weeks to months of the manufacturing date. The loss of potency is related to time, temperature, the concentration of the allergen, the preservative used, and the presence of interfering substance. Outdated extracts should not be used; and the use of allergens close to their expiration date is also questionable, since these antigens are not at their original potency.

Extract potency is greatly affected by the preservative used. Extracts preserved with 50 percent glycerin are the most stable, while phenol-preserved extracts are the least so. Preservation with 10 percent glycerin or 0.03 percent human serum albumin (HSA) gives intermediate results. Since glycerinated extracts can cause false-positive skin test reactions, they are not recommended for use in skin testing in veterinary medicine. HSA allergens have not been studied in animals.

The decay of phenol-preserved extracts is affected by time, temperature, and the concentration of the allergen. Old extracts lose biologic potency, and the degradation products formed can be irritating. Refrigeration is the primary retardant of decay. Periodic exposure of antigens, especially those diluted to skin test strength, to room temperature increases the potency loss. Within a year, diluted extracts preserved with phenol can lose 50 percent of their original activity.

Proteolytic enzymes that are naturally present in the vaccine or that are introduced by bacterial contamination will lower its potency. Contaminated vaccine also can be dangerous, so any vaccine that changes physical characteristics should be discarded. Very concentrated allergens (1:10 W/V or 40,000 PNU/ml) tend to precipitate when they are stored over three to six months. Precipitated extracts are not as potent and may be antigenically different, so they should be discarded.

STANDARDIZATION OF ALLERGENIC EXTRACTS

Because of variations in collection techniques, extraction techniques, and so forth, the composition of allergy extracts is very variable and, unfortunately, no uniform method of standardization exists. Only when an accurate measurement of biologic potency is available will standardization become practicable.

In the United States, extracts are sold either on a weight to volume (W/V) basis or with the concentration indicated as protein nitrogen units (PNU) per milliiter. The W/V concentration is determined by dividing the weight of the defatted allergen by the volume of the diluent. For example, one gram of allergen diluted with 1000 milliliters of diluent yields a 1:1000 solution. The PNU concentration is determined by extracting the protein from the allergen with phosphotungstic acid. By definition, 1 milligram of protein is equal to 100,000 PNU.

Neither method gives a true indication of biologic potency. With the PNU method, one would have to assume that all proteins present are antigenically active and that there are no nonprotein antigens. Neither of these assumptions is true. In the W/V method, the amount of nonprotein material is unknown. If significant amounts of nonprotein material were present, the extract probably would be less potent than the concentration indicated. Neither method addresses the problems of the variability of antigenic determinants in various batches of crude allergens or the effect of extraction on the antigens.

A formula exists to estimate the PNU concentration of a weight/volume extract. One milliliter of a 1:50 W/V solution should contain approximately 10,000 PNU. According to this formula, 1 milliliter of a 1:1000 W/V solution should contain 500 PNU. Many investigators have indicated that house dust is too irritating to dogs to allow for skin testing at 1000 PNU/ml. Concentrations at or below 250 PNU/ml are necessary to limit the number of false-positive reactions. Scott, however, found a low incidence of false-positive reactions to house dust when he tested dogs at 1:1000 W/V, so he continued to use this concentration. The PNU concentration of one batch of house dust allergen was determined by the allergy laboratory and was found to be 200 PNU/ml and not the 500 PNU/ml that the formula predicted. If previous batches of house dust antigen were equally dilute, Scott would have been testing dogs with concentrations in line with those suggested by other authors.

Gel diffusion techniques, histamine release assays, and radioallergosorbent tests (RAST) are all used to measure antigenic potency of extracts. Although the RAST is not commonly used, the results seem to be a reliable indication of the potency of the extract. Until the RAST concentration or some other more precise method of potency determination is available, the authors suggest that allergens be purchased on the PNU/ml basis to avoid any inconsistencies that the W/V method may introduce.

Ultimately, the true test of biologic potency is the skin test reactivity of an allergen. Batches that give fewer or greater numbers of reactions than expected probably have a concentration different from that indicated.

INDIVIDUAL VERSUS GROUPED ALLERGENS

Allergens can be purchased as individual extracts or in stock mixtures. The use of mixtures for skin testing is controversial even though it decreases the number of skin tests per animal and also decreases the cost of the allergens. The reliability of the test results can be questionable. Scott reported poor correlation between mixed and individual allergens when he compared molds, epidermals, and weeds. The tendency was for his and also the authors' patients to react to the individual allergen but not to the group antigen. He did find that mixed grass, mixed ragweed, and mixed dust antigens were satisfactory, but one author (LMR) disagrees. On the other hand, Nesbitt found that the correlation rate between individual and mixed antigens varied from 60 to 75 percent. Unlike Scott, he found a higher reactivity to mixed antigens than to individual allergens.

Group allergens are prepared by mixing small amounts of each ingredient in the same vial. One milliliter of a five-allergen mixture at a strength of 1000 PNU/ml would contain 200 PNU of each antigen. At skin testing, the animal would be injected with 10 PNU of each allergen instead of 50 PNU, which would be the amount used for individual allergens. If more than five antigens are mixed together, the concentration of each allergen would be even lower.

Stock mixtures containing all allergens are not available. If only mixtures are used when testing the animal, some important allergens may be overlooked. Assuming that the mixtures contained all of the pertinent allergens, skin test reactions must be evaluated carefully. A negative reaction to a mixture could indicate that the animal was not sensitive to any of the allergens or that the concentrations of the individual antigens were too low to cause a reaction. Schick's data show that approximately 50 percent of atopic dogs that react to house dust at a strength of 25 PNU/ml will not react to extracts at a strength of 2.5 PNU/ml. The minimum amount of allergen necessary to cause skin test reactivity is unknown and would vary with the dog and the allergen used. True positive reactions would indicate that the animal is sensitive to one or more of the antigens in the mixture. If the animal is truly sensitive to all of the antigens, the use of that mixture for immunotherapy is valid. If the animal is sensitive only to one or several of the allergens, the concentration of the important allergens in the vaccine would be lowered by the nonreactive substances.

If all allergens were antigenically unique, the use of large mixtures would be very questionable. Since some allergens share common antigens, some mixtures may be valid. Stock mixtures that contain very dissimilar allergens such as house dust, epidermals, and mixed insects should not be used. Mixtures should include only similar antigens.

Mixed grass antigen probably is the most valid mixture since most grasses except Bermuda share at least one common antigen. Because rye grass, meadow fescue, orchard grass, and velvet grass share two common antigens, these grasses should show significant cross-reactivity. Ideally, grasses should be tested for individually. If the circumstances necessitate the use of mixtures, one or two mixed suburban grass antigens should be used. In those areas where timothy or Bermuda grasses are prevalent, these allergens should be used separately.

The cross-reactivity of trees, weeds, and molds is questionable. Trees or weeds within the same family may cross-react, while species within the same genus should be even more similar. Ragweed pollens share antigens, so mixed ragweed antigen should give valid results. Similarly, mixtures of rough pigweed, spiny pigweed, careless weed, and Palmer's amaranth; lamb's quarter, Jerusalem oak, and Mexican tea; yellow dock and sheep sorrel; rough marsh elder and burweed marsh elder; allscale, lenscale, and wingscale; and mugwort, wormwood, costal sage, and big sagebrush should be valid since these weeds are grouped by family and genus. Because plants of the *Ambrosia, Iva,* and *Xanthium* genera produce similar pollens and share some ragweed Antigen E activity, mixtures of ragweed, cocklebur, and marsh elder could be valid. Members of the Chenopodiaceae and Amaranthaceae families are thought to be similar, so mixtures of lamb's quarter, Mexican tea, Russian thistle, burning bush (Kochia), and pigweed may be valid.

Nesbitt correlated the number of positive and negative skin test reactions for four weed pairs and found a correlation of 59 percent for lamb's quarter and pigweed, 65 percent for mixed ragweed and rough marsh elder, 66 percent for mixed ragweed and cocklebur, and 62 percent for mixed ragweed and mugwort. These data show that weeds of different genera do not completely cross-react and that weeds from different families (lamb's quarter and pigweed) cross-react less than weeds from the same family (ragweed, marsh elder, cocklebur, and mugwort). Based upon these and other data, the authors do not believe that the use of mixtures of weeds from different genera is reliable enough. Weeds should be tested individually or as mixtures from the same genus.

The use of tree or mold mixtures should follow along the same line. Mixtures of different species from the same genus should be most cross-reactive, while mixtures from different families should be least reactive. Nesbitt tested a mold mixture of four fungi, two of which were from the Dematiaceae family while the other two were from the Moniliaceae family. When he compared the results of the mixed and individual allergens, his correlation ranged from 63 to 65 percent. If the two members of each family were completely cross-reactive, one would expect a higher correlation rate.

From the foregoing discussion, it should be apparent that testing with individual allergens should give more accurate results. When mixtures are to be used, members from the same genus should be grouped together. Mixtures of allergens from the same family but from different genera may not be reliable. The botanic classification of important pollens is shown in Tables 3–1 to 3–3 on pages 67 to 75. These tables represent a compilation of the information supplied to the authors by Center Laboratories, Hollister-Stier, and Greer Laboratories, Inc. Ideally, an animal that reacts to a mixed antigen should be tested for the individual components of the mixture to determine which allergens are significant. This obviously negates the advantages of using mixed allergens. Nesbitt noted a trend that immunotherapy with vaccines containing individual mold, grass, and tree allergens gave better results in dogs than immunotherapy with vaccines containing mixtures. Nonreactive allergens in mixtures will decrease the concentration of the important allergens in the vaccine and may make the vaccine less effective.

ALLERGENS OF SIGNIFICANCE IN VETERINARY MEDICINE

It is virtually impossible to compare the data from one veterinary dermatologist with the next since many different allergens, allergen concentrations, and techniques are used. Tables 3–4 to 3–8 (pages 76 to 80) show the incidence of skin test reactivity of dogs as found by four different investigations. Since these studies only cover a limited geographic area, the reader is referred to the next chapter for a more precise description of important pollen allergens.

TABLE 3–1. Botanical Classification of Grasses of the Gramineae Family

GENUS (COMMON NAME)	SPECIES	COMMON NAME	SYNONYMS	POLLINATION PERIOD
Agrostis	*Tenuis*	Colonial Bentgrass	Creeping Bent	Late Spring
(Bentgrasses)	*Alba*	Redtop	Herd's Grass	Summer
	Dactylon	Bermuda	Devil, Scutch, Wire Grass	Spring, Summer, Fall
Cyndon	*Compressa*	Canada	English Bluegrass Wire Grass	Summer
Poa (Bluegrasses)				
	Pratensis	Kentucky	June Grass, Meadow Grass	Summer
	Sandbergii	Sandberg		Late Spring and Summer
Bromus	*Rigidus*	Broncho	Ripgut	Late Spring
(Bromegrasses)	*Carinatus*	California Bromegrass		Late Spring/Early Summer
	Secalinus	Cheat	Chess, Rye-Brome Cock-grass	Summer
	Inermis	Bromegrass	Hungarian Bromegrass	Summer
	Unioloides	Southern Chess	Soft Chess	Summer
Phalaris	*Canariensis*	Canary Grass		Late Spring
(Canary Grasses)	*Arundinacea*	Reed Canary		Summer
	Minor	Small Canary	Mediterranean	Spring
Festuca	*Elatior*	Meadow Fescue	Tall Fescue, Dover Grass	Summer
(Fescues)	*Rubra*	Red Fescue		Summer
Sorghum	*Halepense*	Johnson Grass	Evergreen Millet	Summer
	Vulgare var sudanense	Sudan Grass		Summer

Table continued on following page

TABLE 3–1. Botanical Classification of Grasses of the Gramineae Family *Continued*

GENUS (COMMON NAME)	SPECIES	COMMON NAME	SYNONYMS	POLLINATION PERIOD
Koeleria	*Cristata*	Koeler's Grass	June Grass, Western June Grass	Summer
Avena	*Sativa*	Cultivated Oat		Late Spring
(Oats)	*Barbata*	Slender Wild Oat		Spring
	Fatua	Wild Oat		Spring and Early Summer
Dactylis	*Glomerata*	Orchard Grass	Dew Grass, Hard Grass, Cocksfoot	Late Spring/Early Summer
Elymus	*Triticoides*	Alkali Rye	Beardless Wildrye	Late Spring
(Wild Ryes)	*Cinereus*	Giant Wildrye		Late Spring/Early Summer
	Glaucus	Western Wildrye	Blue Wildrye	Early Summer
Lolium	*Multiflorum*	Italian Ryegrass	Ryegrass	Summer
(Rye Grasses)	*Perenne*	Perennial Rye Grass	English Rye	Summer
Distichlis	*Stricata*	Salt Grass	Alkali Grass	Summer
Anthoxanthum	*Odoratum*	Sweet Vernalgrass		Spring
Phleum	*Pratense*	Timothy	Herd's Grass	Late Spring/Summer
Holcus	*Lanatus*	Velvet Grass	Soft Grass, Feather Grass	Summer
Triticum	*Aestivum*	Wheat		Early Summer
Agropyron	*Repens*	Quackgrass	Quitchgrass	Early Summer
(Wheatgrasses)	*Smithii*	Western Wheatgrass	Bluejoint, Bluestem	Summer

TABLE 3–2. Botanical Classification of Trees of Allergenic Significance

FAMILY	GENUS	SPECIES	COMMON NAME	SYNONYMS	POLLINATION PERIOD
Aceraceae	*Acer*	*Negundo*	Box Elder	Ash-leaved Maple Cut-leaved Maple	Spring
	Acer	*Macrophyllum*	Coast Maple	Broad-leaved Maple	Spring
	Acer	*Saccharum*	Hard Maple	Sugar, Black, Rock	Spring
	Acer	*Rubrum*	Red Maple	Scarlet, Swamp, White	Early Spring
	Acer	*Saccharinum*	Silver Maple	River, Soft, Swamp	Late Winter
Betulaceae	*Alnus*	*Sinuata*	Sitka Alder	Wavy-leaved	Spring and Early Summer
	Alnus	*Tenuifolia*	Slender Alder	Mountain	Spring
	Alnus	*Rugosa*	Tag Alder	Hoary, Speckled	Early Spring
	Alnus	*Rhombifolia*	White Alder	Alder	Early Spring
	Betula	*Papyrifera*	Paper Birch	Canoe	Spring
	Betula	*Nigra*	Red Birch	River, Water	Spring
	Betula	*Occidentalis*	Spring Birch	California, Black, Mountain	Spring
	Betula	*Pendula*	White Birch	European White	Spring
	Corylus	*Americana*	American Hazelnut	Filbert, Hazel	Early Spring
	Corylus	*Californica*	California Hazelnut	California Hazel	Early Spring

Table continued on following page

TABLE 3–2. Botanical Classification of Trees of Allergenic Significance *Continued*

FAMILY	GENUS	SPECIES	COMMON NAME	SYNONYMS	POLLINATION PERIOD
Fagaceae	*Fagus*	*Grandifolia*	Beech		Spring
	Quercus	*Macrocarpa*	Burr Oak	Mossy Cup	Spring
	Quercus	*Kelloggii*	California Black Oak	Kellogg's Oak	Spring
	Quercus	*Agrifolia*	Coast Live Oak	Live Oak	Spring
	Quercus	*Gambelii*	Gambel Oak	Rocky Mountain White Oak	Spring
	Quercus	*Garryana*	Garry's Oak	Oregon, Western White	Spring
	Quercus	*Stellata*	Post Oak	Iron	Spring
	Quercus	*Rubra*	Red Oak		Spring
	Quercus	*Dumosa*	Scrub Oak		Spring
	Quercus	*Lobata*	Valley Oak	White Oak	Spring
	Quercus	*Virginiana*	Virginia Live Oak	Eastern Live, Texas Live	Spring
	Quercus	*Alba*	White Oak		Spring
Hammelidaceae	*Liquidambar*	*Styraciflua*	Sweetgum	Liquidambar	Late Spring
Juglandaceae	*Carya*	*Pecan*	Pecan		Spring
	Carya	*Ovata*	Shagbark Hickory	Shag	Late Spring
	Carya	*Tomentosa*	White Hickory	Mockernut	Late Spring
	Juglans	*Nigra*	Black Walnut		Spring
	Juglans	*Regia*	English Walnut	Persian	Spring
	Juglans	*Hindsii*	California Black Walnut		Spring
	Juglans	*Californica*	Southern California Black Walnut		Early Spring

Leguminosae	*Acacia*	Spp.	Acacia	Cassie, Wattle	Late Winter, Spring
	Prosopis	*Juliflora*	Mesquite	Honey Mesquite, Honey Locust	Spring and Summer
Moraceae	*Morus*	Spp.	Mulberry		Spring
Myrtaceae	*Eucalyptus*	*Globulus*	Eucalyptus	Gum Tree	All Seasons
Oleaceae	*Fraxinus*	*Velutina*	Arizona Ash		Spring
	Fraxinus	*Pennsylvanica*	Green Ash		Spring
	Fraxinus	*Americana*	White Ash		Spring
	Olea	*Europaea*	Olive		Late Spring
	Liqustrum	*Vulgare*	Privet		Late Spring
Pinaceae	*Juniperus*	*Asheii*	Mountain Cedar	Juniper, Mexican, Rock	Winter
	Juniperus	*Virginiana*	Red Cedar	Red Savin, Carolina Cedar, Pencil Wood	Early Spring
	Juniperus	*Occidentalis*	Western Juniper	Juniper	Spring
	Cupressus	*Arizonica*	Arizona Cypress		Early Spring
	Cupressus	*Sempervirens*	Italian Cypress		Late Winter
	Cupressus	*Macrocarpa*	Monterey Cypress		Spring
	Pseudotsuga	*Menziesii*	Douglas Fir	Douglas Spruce, Oregon Pine	Spring
	Pinus	*Contorta*	Lodgepole Pine	Scrub Pine	Late Spring
	Pinus	*Ponderosa*	Yellow Pine	Bull, Ponderosa	Late Spring
	Pinus	*Strobus*	Eastern White Pine		Late Spring
	Pinus	*Monticola*	Western White Pine		Late Spring

Table continued on following page

TABLE 3–2. Botanical Classification of Trees of Allergenic Significance *Continued*

FAMILY	GENUS	SPECIES	COMMON NAME	SYNONYMS	POLLINATION PERIOD
Platanaceae	*Platanus*	*Racemosa*	California Sycamore	Planetree, Western Sycamore	Early Spring
	Platanus	*Occidentalis*	Eastern Sycamore	Planetree, Button-ball, Buttonwood	Spring
	Platanus	*Acerifolia*	Maple Leaf Sycamore	London Planetree, "Oriental" Sycamore	Spring
Salicaceae	*Populus*	*Tremuloides*	Aspen	Poplar, Aspen, Quaking Aspen	Spring
	Populus	*Balsamifera*	Balsam		Early Spring
	Populus	*Trichocarpa*	Black Cottonwood		Early Spring
	Populus	*Deltoides*	Common Cottonwood	Necklace Poplar	Early Spring
	Populus	*Fremontii*	Fremont Cottonwood	California	Early Spring
	Populus	*Alba*	White Poplar	Abele, Silver	Early Spring
	Salix	Spp.	Willow		Late Winter, Spring
Taxodiaceae	*Sequoia*	*Sempervirens*	Redwood		Spring
Tiliaceae	*Tilia*	*Americana*	Linden	Basswood, Whitewood	Spring
Ulmaceae	*Ulmus*	*Americana*	American Elm	White Elm	Early Spring
	Ulmus	*Pumila*	Evergreen Elm	Chinese	Early Spring
	Ulmus	*Parvifolia*	Chinese Elm	Evergreen Elm, Silver Elm	Early Spring
	Celtis	*Occidentalis*	Hackberry	False Elm, Sugarberry, Hoop Ash	Spring

TABLE 3–3. Botanical Classification of Weeds of Allergenic Significance

FAMILY	GENUS	SPECIES	COMMON NAME	SYNONYMS	POLLINATION PERIOD
Amaranthaceae	*Amaranthus*	*Palmeri*	Careless Weed		Summer
	Amaranthus	*Retroflexus*	Rough Redroot, Pigweed	Rough Pigweed, Green Amaranth	Summer
	Amaranthus	*Spinosus*	Spiny Pigweed		Summer
	Amaranthus	*Tamariscinus*	Waterhemp	Western Waterhemp	Late Summer
Chenopodiaceae	*Bassia*	*Hyssopifolia*	Bassia	Five-hook Bassia	Summer
	Beta	*Vulgaris*	Sugar Beet		Late Spring and Summer
	Sarcobatus	*Vermiculatus*	Greasewood	Chico	Late Spring/Early Summer
	Allenrolfea	*Occidentalis*	Iodine Bush	Burroweed	Summer
	Kochia	*Scoparia*	Kochia	Burning Bush, Summer Cypress, Fireweed, Belvedere	Summer
	Chenopodium	*Album*	Lamb's Quarter	White Pigweed, Pigweed	Spring and Summer
	Chenopodium	*Ambrosioides*	Mexican Tea	Wormseed	Late Summer/Early Fall
	Salicornia	*Ambigua*	Pickleweed	Grasswort, Samphire	Late Spring and Summer
	Salsola	*Kali*	Russian Thistle	Tumbleweed, Saltwort	Summer
	Atriplex	*Polycarpa*	Allscale	Desert Sage	Late Summer
	Atriplex	*Wrightii*	Annual Saltbush		Summer
	Atriplex	*Serenana*	Bractscale		Summer
	Atriplex	*Lentiformis*	Lenscale	Quailbrush	Late Summer
	Atriplex	*Confertifolia*	Sheepfat	Shadscale, Spiny Saltbush	Late Spring/Early Summer

Table continued on following page

TABLE 3–3. Botanical Classification of Weeds of Allergenic Significance *Continued*

FAMILY	GENUS	SPECIES	COMMON NAME	SYNONYMS	POLLINATION PERIOD
Chenopodiaceae (*Continued*)	*Atriplex*	*Argentea expansa*	Silverscale	Silver Orach	Summer
	Atriplex	*Patula hastata*	Spearscale		Summer
	Atriplex	*Canescens*	Wingscale	Shadscale	Summer
	Eurotia	*Lanata*	Winter Fat	Sweet Sage	Late Spring
Compositae	*Balsamorhiza*	*Sagittata*	Balsam Root		Spring
	Iva	*Xanthifolia*	Burweed Marshelder	Prairie Ragweed	Summer
	Iva	*Ciliata*	Marshelder	Rough Marshelder	Summer
	Iva	*Angustifolia*	Narrowleaf Marshelder	Small-flowered Marshelder	Late Spring and Summer
	Xanthium	*Commune*	Cocklebur	Clotbur	Late Summer
	Taraxacum	*Officinale*	Dandelion		Spring and Summer
	Solidago	Spp.	Goldenrod		Late Summer/Early Fall
	Ambrosia	*Artemisiifolia*	Short Ragweed	Low, common	Late Summer/Fall
	Ambrosia	*Trifida*	Giant Ragweed	Tall	Late Summer/Fall
	Ambrosia	*Bidentata*	Southern Ragweed		Late Summer
	Ambrosia	*Psilostachya*	Western Ragweed		Late Summer/Early Fall
	Franseria	*Acanthicarpa*	False Ragweed	Beachbur, Beach Sandbur	Spring and Summer
	Franseria	*Dumosa*	Desert Ragweed	Burrobush, Burroweed, Desert Bursage	Spring
	Ambrosia	*Deltoidea*	Rabbit Bush	Canyon Ragweed, Arizona Bursage	Spring

	Dicoria	*Canescens*	Silver Ragweed	Dicoria	Fall
	Artemisia	*Annua*	Annual Sagebrush	Sagewort, Annual Wormwort	Summer
	Artemisia	*Tridentata*	Common Sagebrush	Mountain Sagebrush	Late Summer and Fall
	Artemisia	*Dracunculus*	Green Sagebrush	Dragon Sagewort, Indian Hair Tonic	Summer
	Artemisia	*Vulgaris*	Mugwort	California Mugwort	Summer
	Artemisia	*Frigida*	Pasture Sagebrush	Carpet Sage, Prairie Sage, Estafiata	Summer/Early Fall
	Artemisia	*Ludoviciana*	White Sagebrush	Prairie Sagebursh, Wormwood	Late Summer/Early Fall
	Artemisia	*Absinthium*	Wormwood	Sagewort, Absinth Sage	Late Summer
Cruciferae	*Brassica*	*Campestris*	Mustard	Field Mustard	Spring and Summer
Plantaginaceae	*Plantago*	*Major*	Common Plantain	Greater Plantain	Late Spring and Summer
	Plantago	*Lanceolata*	English Plantain	Buckhorn, Ribgrass	Spring and Summer
Polygonaceae	*Rumex*	*Obtusifolius*	Bitter Dock	Broadleaf	Summer
	Rumex	*Acetosella*	Sheep Sorrel	Sorrel Dock, Field Sorrel, Red Sorrel	Late Spring
	Rumex	*Crispus*	Yellow Dock	Curly Dock	Summer
Urticaceae	*Urtica*	*Dioica*	Nettle	Hoary Nettle	Summer

TABLE 3–4. Skin Test Reactivity (%) of Dogs to Grass Antigens

ALLERGEN	NEW YORK[1]	NEW YORK[2]	PACIFIC NORTHWEST[3]	NORTHERN FLORIDA[4]	SOUTHERN FLORIDA[4]	ILLINOIS[4]	NORTH CAROLINA[4]
Mixed	30	53	85	21	39	29	18
June	—	48	—	—	—	—	—
Orchard	—	50	82	—	—	—	—
Timothy	—	47	76	34	46	22	29
Sweet Vernal	—	40	84	—	—	—	—
Red Top	—	44	—	—	—	—	—
Meadow Fescue	—	45	—	—	—	—	—
Bermuda	—	—	—	38	52	21	25
Bahia	—	—	—	45	61	19	29
Johnson	—	—	—	36	37	15	21
Salt	—	—	—	28	19	2	7
Rye	—	67	83	—	—	—	—
Blue	—	—	89	—	—	—	—
Velvet	—	—	76	—	—	—	—

1. Scott, 1981.
2. Nesbitt, 1984.
3. Nesbitt, 1978.
4. Schick, 1986.

TABLE 3–5. Skin Test Reactivity (%) of Dogs to Tree Antigens

ALLERGEN	NEW YORK[1]	NEW YORK[2]	PACIFIC NORTHWEST[3]	NORTHERN FLORIDA[4]	SOUTHERN FLORIDA[4]	ILLINOIS[4]	NORTH CAROLINA[4]
Mixed	27	47	78	—	—	—	—
Ash	—	35	71	—	—	—	—
Birch	—	35	70	—	—	—	—
Beech	—	29	—	21	19	11	14
Elm	—	36	—	21	24	5	11
Hickory	—	39	—	26	30	5	21
Maple	—	29	82	—	—	—	—
Poplar	—	32	—	25	28	4	11
Oak	—	38	78	—	—	—	—
Red Cedar	—	39	—	38	40	13	25
Pine	—	32	—	26	9	9	14
Cottonwood	—	—	73	—	—	—	—
Willow	—	—	79	34	24	12	11
Alder	—	—	79	—	—	—	—
Walnut	—	—	56	30	27	7	21
Hackberry	—	—	—	30	28	15	21
Pecan	—	—	—	38	39	8	32
Palm	—	—	—	38	42	4	21
Live Oak	—	—	—	42	39	4	14
Sycamore	—	—	—	23	28	2	14
Sweet Gum	—	—	—	21	24	0	18
Acacia	—	—	—	32	36	1	14
Mango	—	—	—	17	28	2	7
Red Mulberry	—	—	—	30	36	2	18
Orange	—	—	—	28	48	3	4
Pepper Tree	—	—	—	34	36	2	14
Australian Pine	—	—	—	28	24	2	4

1. Scott, 1981.
2. Nesbitt, 1984.
3. Nesbitt, 1978.
4. Schick, 1986.

TABLE 3–6. Skin Test Reactivity (%) of Dogs to Weed Antigens

ALLERGEN	NEW YORK[1]	NEW YORK[2]	PACIFIC NORTHWEST[3]	NORTHERN FLORIDA[4]	SOUTHERN FLORIDA[4]	ILLINOIS[4]	NORTH CAROLINA[4]
Mixed	—	63	80	—	—	—	—
Lamb's Quarter	10	60	77	47	37	25	29
Cocklebur	13	59	—	34	42	32	32
English Plantain	17	46	75	25	33	22	25
Rough Marsh Elder	10	62	—	42	48	33	32
Sheep Sorrel	17	46	72	38	33	33	32
Pigweed	15	56	80	40	37	22	36
Mugwort	—	52	—	—	—	—	—
Mixed Ragweed	35	59	—	38	39	45	39
Yellow Dock	17	—	78	47	55	33	29
Goldenrod	35	—	—	26	42	20	25
Dog Fennel	—	—	—	32	40	24	36
Baccharis spp.	—	—	—	30	39	14	21
Kochia	17	—	—	43	45	25	36
Dandelion	22	—	76	—	—	—	—

1. Scott, 1981.
2. Nesbitt, 1984.
3. Nesbitt, 1978.
4. Schick, 1986.

TABLE 3–7. Skin Test Reactivity (%) of Dogs to Fungal Antigens

ALLERGEN	NEW YORK[1]	NEW YORK[2]	PACIFIC NORTHWEST[3]	NORTHERN FLORIDA[4]	SOUTHERN FLORIDA[4]	ILLINOIS[4]	NORTH CAROLINA[4]
Mixed	—	43	88	—	—	—	—
Cladosporium (Hormodendum)	15	35	80	—	—	—	—
Alternaria	25	37	79	15	15	21	18
Aspergillus	15	42	—	15	19	27	11
Penicillium	15	47	84	17	24	24	18
Botrytis	20	33	—	—	—	—	—
Phoma	35	35	—	—	—	—	—
Epicoccum	8	32	—	—	—	—	—
Mucor	35	39	—	—	—	—	—
Aerobasidium (Pullularia)	40	42	—	—	—	—	—
Helminthosporium	42	30	—	—	—	—	—
Curvularia	—	38	—	—	—	—	—
Rhodotorula	—	40	—	—	—	—	—
Fusarium	42	37	—	—	—	—	—
Rhizopus	20	42	—	—	—	—	—
Stemphyllium	8	—	—	—	—	—	—

1. Scott, 1981.
2. Nesbitt, 1984.
3. Nesbitt, 1978.
4. Schick, 1986.

TABLE 3–8. Skin Test Reactivity (%) of Dogs to Environmental Antigens

ALLERGEN	NEW YORK[1]	NEW YORK[2]	PACIFIC NORTHWEST[3]	NORTHERN FLORIDA[4]	SOUTHERN FLORIDA[4]	ILLINOIS[4]	NORTH CAROLINA[4]
House Dust	35	64	71	68	49	34	39
House Dust Mite	—	—	—	62	46	34	46
Mixed Epidermals	30	76	—	—	—	—	—
Cat Epithelium	30	71	67	36	18	1	18
Dog Epithelium	—	74	56	—	—	—	—
Horse Epithelium	—	65	75	—	—	—	—
Human Epithelium	50	—	17	—	—	—	—
Mixed Feathers	35	76	51	11	15	25	32
Wool	35	59	63	21	24	27	32
Kapok	48	50	84	23	22	24	21
Cottonseed	25	53	—	—	—	—	—
Tobacco	38	—	28	—	—	—	—
Newsprint	30	—	—	—	—	—	—

1. Scott, 1981.
2. Nesbitt, 1984.
3. Nesbitt, 1978.
4. Schick, 1986.

4 Allergy Testing

INTRODUCTION

Allergy testing is used to confirm the tentative diagnosis of atopic disease but, more importantly, to identify the offending allergens. Once the allergens are identified, specific therapies of avoidance, immunotherapy, or both can be initiated. Since avoidance is rarely practical, allergy testing should be conducted only when immunotherapy would be appropriate. If symptomatic treatment is the only modality to be used, allergy testing is a needless expense with no therapeutic benefit.

Both in vivo and in vitro methods of allergy testing are available. In vitro testing involves the serum measurement of immunoreactants involved in the allergic reaction. In vivo allergy testing revolves around the induction of a small-scale allergic reaction by the intentional exposure of the patient to a minute amount of allergen. In vitro testing is discussed later in this chapter.

In vivo allergy testing can be done via the conjunctiva, skin, or nasal or bronchial mucosa. In the clinical situation, the skin is the only practical site, as it is readily accessible, easily observed, and easily tested, and a large number of tests can be performed safely at one time. Skin test reactivity only indicates skin sensitivity. The clinical significance of test reactions must be determined by their correlation with the patient's history.

ALLERGEN PURCHASE

Allergens can be purchased from various laboratories in different strengths and volumes. Since there is no standardization of allergens among laboratories, allergens should be purchased from the same laboratory, and the allergens used for skin testing should also be used for immunotherapy.

When the decision to conduct skin testing is made, one must also decide whether to order concentrated or skin test–strength antigens. If skin test–strength antigens are purchased, separate vaccines for immunotherapy must be purchased from the antigen supplier. Because of government sterility requirements, the delivery of custom-made vaccines will take at least one month.

The purchase of concentrated antigens gives veterinarians the flexibility of making their own skin test antigens as well as the vaccines for immunotherapy. Concentrated allergens come in different strengths and volumes. The higher the concentration and the larger the volume purchased, the lower the cost on a PNU/ml basis. Very concentrated allergens tend to precipitate out and should not be purchased unless the vial is to be used within six months. A concentration of 20,000 PNU/ml is most appropriate.

The decision to buy diluted or concentrated allergens is often an economic one. Allergens must be used before their expiration dates. If the number of patients to receive a hyposensitization vaccine is small, the allergens may expire before they are used. In this case the veterinarian will have to absorb the cost, or the cost of each vaccine will be very high. It is impossible to calculate the exact number of cases needed to reach the breakeven point, but if fewer than 15 vaccines are to be made each year, it would not be economical to purchase concentrated allergens. If between 15 and 30 vaccines are made each year, the cost of the allergens will be recovered with a small profit for the veterinarian. As the number of yearly vaccines increases, the cost per vaccine decreases to the point at which the vaccine can cost one-half of that charged by the antigen supplier.

SELECTION OF TEST ANTIGENS

In the United States, approximately 425 nonfood allergy extracts are commercially available. Obviously it is impossible to test for all of these allergens. Although certain allergens are not found in some floristic zones and can easily be eliminated from consideration, the number of allergens remaining will still be excessive.

Figure 4–1 shows a map of the botanic or floristic zones of the United States as supplied to the authors by Greer Laboratories, Inc.; Tables 4–1 through 4–10 list important pollen allergens found in each region. The data in Tables 4–1 through 4–10 were tabulated from materials supplied by Center Laboratories, Hollister-Stier, and Greer Laboratories, Inc. These lists should not be considered all inclusive or exclusive. As each region is quite large, some pollens are not found in all states. For example, Bermuda grass is listed in region 1, but it is restricted to the southern portions of Pennsylvania and New Jersey. Even in one area of a particular zone, the prevalent pollens can vary greatly, as the degree and nature of urban development affect the types and numbers of plants. In agricultural areas, cultivated crops of corn, rye, barley, oats, wheat, alfalfa, castor beans, and sugar beets may produce significant allergens for pets. The allergy laboratories and the personnel of the local weather bureau, health department, medical school, or veterinary college can aid in antigen selection. Perhaps the best source of accurate

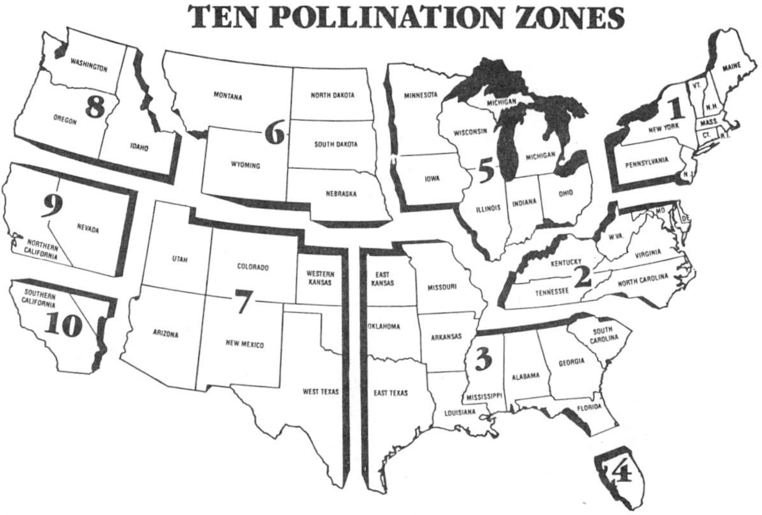

FIGURE 4–1. Botanic zones of the United States. (Courtesy of Greer Labs Inc., Lenoir, N.C.)

local information is the human allergist, as pollens that are important in humans are probably important in animals. Important local fungal antigens, such as barn molds, can be identified by exposing malt agar culture plates to the air for one hour. Standard mycologic techniques are used to identify all growths.

Since there are vast numbers of regional allergens, any skin test set will be incomplete but, hopefully, will include all or most of the important allergens. Because the botanic and climatic conditions in an area change, the importance of a particular allergen can also change. All skin test results should be kept in a tabular form and reviewed at least yearly. Allergens with a low incidence of reactivity (approximately 5 percent) are not of major importance and can be replaced with a new allergen. The elimination of an allergen with a low reactivity means that an important allergen will be missed in a small number of animals.

Tables 4–11 and 4–12 list the allergens the authors presently use in their skin testing. Not all animals necessarily will be tested for all allergens. Animals with summer allergies may not have to be tested for indoor antigens, while perennially allergic dogs are tested for all appropriate allergens.

Obviously, the authors use a significantly different number of allergens for testing. These sets were developed over a number of years and reflect the nature of the practices, the importance of the various allergens in each area, and a number of other factors. As a

TABLE 4–1. Pollens of Importance—Area 1

MAINE, NEW HAMPSHIRE, VERMONT, MASSACHUSETTS, RHODE ISLAND, CONNECTICUT, NEW YORK, NEW JERSEY, PENNSYLVANIA		
GRASSES	**TREES/SHRUBS**	**WEEDS**
Bermuda	Alder, Tag	Cocklebur
Blue, Kentucky	Ash, White	Dock, Yellow
Brome, Smooth	Ash, Green	Goldenrod
Fescue, Meadow	Aspen	Kochia
Johnson	Beech	Lamb's Quarter
Orchard	Birch, White	Marsh Elder
Quack	Birch, Cherry	Mugwort
Red Top	Birch, Red	Pigweed, Rough
Rye, Perennial	Birch, Yellow	Pigweed, Spiny
Rye, Italian	Birch, Paper	Plantain, English
Sweet Vernal	Box Elder	Ragweed, Giant
Timothy	Cedar, Red	Ragweed, Short
Velvet	Cottonwood, Common	Sorrel, Sheep
	Elm, American	Wormwood
	Hackberry	
	Hazelnut, American	
	Hickory, White	
	Hickory, Shagbark	
	Hickory, Shellbark	
	Maple, Red	
	Maple, Sugar	
	Maple, Silver	
	Mulberry, Red	
	Oak, Black	
	Oak, Bur	
	Oak, Red	
	Oak, White	
	Pine, Eastern White	
	Sweet Gum	
	Sycamore, American	
	Walnut, Black	
	Willow	

general rule, satisfactory information can be obtained with 25 to 30 well-selected allergens. The beginner should select approximately 20 of the most important local pollens (grasses, weeds, and trees) and add four or five molds. House dust, important epidermals (human, cat, and the like), and mixed feathers should be included as well as a positive and negative control. As one becomes familiar with this initial test set and with allergy testing in general, shortcomings of the test antigens will become obvious and allergens can be added or dropped as needed. With a new allergy test set, the test results should be reviewed every few months for the first year to make sure that the concentration of the antigens is correct and

TABLE 4–2. Pollens of Importance—Area 2

MARYLAND, DELAWARE, DISTRICT OF COLUMBIA, VIRGINIA, WEST VIRGINIA, KENTUCKY, NORTH CAROLINA, TENNESSEE

GRASSES	TREES/SHRUBS	WEEDS
Bermuda	Alder, Tag	Cocklebur
Blue, Kentucky	Ash, White	Dock, Yellow
Brome, Smooth	Ash, Green	Dog Fennel
Fescue, Meadow	Aspen	Goldenrod
Johnson	Bayberry	Lamb's Quarter
Orchard	Beech	Marsh Elder
Quack	Birch, Red	Mugwort
Red Top	Box Elder	Pigweed, Rough
Rye, Perennial	Cedar, Red	Pigweed, Spiny
Rye, Italian	Cottonwood, Common	Plantain, English
Sweet Vernal	Cypress, Bald	Ragweed, Giant
Timothy	Elm, American	Ragweed, Short
Velvet	Hackberry	Sorrel, Sheep
	Hazelnut, American	Wormwood
	Hickory, White	
	Hickory, Shagbark	
	Hickory, Shellbark	
	Maple, Red	
	Maple, Sugar	
	Maple, Silver	
	Mulberry, Red	
	Mulberry, White	
	Mulberry, Paper	
	Oak, Black	
	Oak, Red	
	Oak, Water	
	Oak, Virginia Live	
	Oak, White	
	Oak, Post	
	Pecan	
	Pine, Virginia Scrub	
	Pine, Loblolly	
	Pine, Shortleaf	
	Sweet Gum	
	Sycamore, American	
	Walnut, Black	
	Willow	

that the testing technique is not causing false-negative or false-positive reactions.

Since the number of test allergens is limited, it is tempting to use mixtures. Scott reported a good correlation between the results obtained with mixed and individual allergens for grasses, ragweed, and house dust but a poor correlation for mixed molds, mixed epidermals, and mixed weeds. He found that dogs that had negative

TABLE 4–3. Pollens of Importance—Area 3

South Carolina, Georgia, Northern Florida, Alabama, Mississippi, Louisiana, Arkansas, East Texas, Oklahoma, East Kansas, Missouri		
GRASSES	**TREES/SHRUBS**	**WEEDS**
Bahia	Alder, Tag	Careless Weed
Bermuda	Ash, White	Cocklebur
Blue, Kentucky	Ash, Green	Dock, Yellow
Brome	Bayberry	Dog Fennel
Fescue, Meadow	Beech	Goldenrod
Johnson	Birch, Red	Kochia
Orchard	Box Elder	Lamb's Quarter
Quack	Cedar, Red	Marsh Elder
Red Top	Cottonwood, Common	Pigweed, Rough
Rye, Perennial	Cypress, Bald	Pigweed, Spiny
Rye, Italian	Elm, Cedar	Plantain, English
Sweet Vernal	Elm, American	Ragweed, Giant
Timothy	Hackberry	Ragweed, Short
Velvet	Hazelnut, American	Ragweed, Southern
	Hickory, White	Sorrel, Sheep
	Hickory, Shagbark	Water Hemp, Western
	Hickory, Shellbark	
	Maple, Red	
	Maple, Sugar	
	Maple, Silver	
	Mesquite	
	Mulberry, Red	
	Mulberry, White	
	Mulberry, Paper	
	Oak, White	
	Oak, Post	
	Oak, Red	
	Oak, Black	
	Oak, Water	
	Oak, Virginia Live	
	Pecan	
	Pine, Virginia Scrub	
	Pine, Loblolly	
	Pine, Shortleaf	
	Sweet Gum	
	Sycamore, American	
	Walnut, Black	
	Willow	

reactions to the mixed antigen could show positive reactions to one or more components of the mixture, if the allergens were tested individually. Nesbitt studied this point more extensively and found dissimilar results. In general, he found more reactivity with the mixed antigens than he did with the individual allergens. By correlating the percentage of reactivity for the mixed and individual

TABLE 4–4. Pollens of Importance—Area 4

South Florida		
GRASSES	**TREES/SHRUBS**	**WEEDS**
Bahia	Bayberry	Baccharis
Bermuda	Box Elder	Cocklebur
Johnson	Hackberry	Dock, Yellow
Rye, Italian	Maple, Red	Dog Fennel
Salt	Melaleuca	Goldenrod
	Mulberry, Red	Lamb's Quarter
	Mulberry, White	Marsh Elder
	Oak, Live	Pigweed, Rough
	Palm	Pigweed, Spiny
	Pine, Australian	Plantain, English
	Pine, Longleaf	Ragweed, Short
	Pine, Slash	Sorrel, Sheep
	Sweet Gum	
	Willow	

allergens, he found a range of 56 to 77 percent for trees, 60 to 67 percent for weeds, 61 to 75 percent for grasses, 61 to 73 percent for molds, and 67 to 77 percent for epidermals. Although these data are very difficult to interpret, they suggest that, depending on the allergen group, mixtures will give reliable results from 56 to 77 percent of the time. The authors believe that these data demonstrate that most mixtures are not reliable enough for use in testing. As was mentioned in the previous chapter, mixtures of grasses and pollens from the same genus may have some applicability, but individual allergens are the most reliable.

Controls

Positive and negative controls are included in each skin test to determine the reactivity of the skin and to grade the skin test reactions. The negative control should be the diluent solution used to dilute the allergens. Most diluents are saline with 0.4 percent phenol added. Although it is rare, the diluent can irritate the skin of some dogs and cause false-positive reactions, which negates the remainder of the test.

The positive control is used to determine the reactivity of the patient's skin. Most allergists use histamine phosphate at a strength of 1:100,000. As mentioned previously, the histamine reactive value may be of some diagnostic significance, so multiple dilutions of histamine may be indicated. Histamine tests the inflammatory response capability of the skin and not the lability of the mast cell. If the histamine reaction is poor, the skin test is invalid as far as negative reactions are concerned. Alternatively, a good histamine

TABLE 4–5. Pollens of Importance—Area 5

Ohio, Michigan, Indiana, Illinois, Wisconsin, Minnesota, Iowa		
GRASSES	**TREES/SHRUBS**	**WEEDS**
Bermuda	Alder, Tag	Cocklebur
Blue, Kentucky	Ash, White	Dandelion
Brome	Ash, Green	Dock, Yellow
Canary, Reed	Aspen	Goldenrod
Johnson	Beech	Kochia
Fescue, Meadow	Birch, Red	Marsh Elder, Burweed
Orchard	Box Elder	Mugwort
Quack	Cedar, Red	Nettle
Rye, Perennial	Cottonwood, Common	Pigweed, Rough
Rye, Italian	Elm, American	Pigweed, Spiny
Sweet Vernal	Hazelnut, American	Ragweed, Giant
Timothy	Hickory, Shagbark	Ragweed, Short
Velvet	Hickory, Shellbark	Ragweed, Western
Western Wheat	Hickory, White	Russian Thistle
	Maple, Red	Sorrel, Sheep
	Maple, Sugar	
	Maple, Silver	
	Mulberry, Red	
	Oak, White	
	Oak, Bur	
	Oak, Red	
	Oak, Black	
	Pecan	
	Pine, Eastern White	
	Pine, Red	
	Sycamore, American	
	Walnut, Black	
	Willow	

reaction does not guarantee that the negative skin test results are valid. The wheals caused by positive reactions to antigens are immunologically mediated and involve mast cell degranulation. Glucocorticoid steroids stabilize cell membranes; this stability can apparently persist for some time.

The compound 48/80 is used by some allergists as a positive control. This compound stimulates mast cell degranulation and mimics immunologic degranulation. Not only is histamine released, but also the other inflammatory mediators are included, so the irritability of the skin is tested in a more natural fashion. A poor response to 48/80 could indicate that the skin has a poor inflammatory response potential or that the mast cells are decreased in number or reactive capability. Because of individual animal variability, a concentration range of 10 to 1000 μg/ml has been suggested.

The ideal positive control would be an antiserum directed against reaginic antibodies (IgE, IgG_d, or both). This antiserum would cause

TABLE 4–6. Pollens of Importance—Area 6

North Dakota, South Dakota, Nebraska, Montana, Wyoming		
GRASSES	**TREES/SHRUBS**	**WEEDS**
Blue, Kentucky	Ash, Green	Cocklebur
Brome	Aspen	Dock, Yellow
Canary, Reed	Box Elder	Kochia
Fescue, Meadow	Cedar, Red	Lamb's Quarter
Grama	Cedar, Rocky Mountain	Marsh Elder, Burweed
Orchard	Cottonwood, Common	Nettle
Quack	Elm, American	Plantain, English
Red Top	Oak, Bur	Povertyweed
Rye, Perennial	Willow	Ragweed, False
Rye, Italian		Ragweed, Giant
Timothy		Ragweed, Short
Western Wheat		Ragweed, Western
Wild rye		Russian Thistle
		Sagebrush, Common
		Sagebrush, White
		Scale, Wing
		Sorrel, Sheep
		Water Hemp, Western

immunologic mast cell degranulation. One author (WHM) used anti-IgE as a positive control and found it to be a better indicator of the reactivity of the dog as compared to histamine. Unfortunately, this antiserum is not commercially available.

Regardless of which positive control is used, if its reaction is poor, the remainder of the skin test is questionable. Positive reactions may be valid, but negative reactions are uninterpretable. With histamine, the maximum reaction occurs 8 to 10 minutes after the injection. With 48/80 or anti-IgE, the wheal reaches maximum size in 12 to 17 minutes. A good positive control reaction should be 15 to 20 mm in diameter.

Test Antigen Concentration

If an allergen is too concentrated, it will cause a reaction in a nonallergic individual. The threshold concentration of an allergen is the maximum concentration at which a minimum (possibly zero) number of nonallergic animals will develop skin test reactions. Accordingly, the concentration of the test allergens should be such that no false-positive reactions occur. If the concentration is too low, allergic patients will not react, thus creating false-negative results. Therefore, the concentration should be adjusted so that the incidence of false-positive reactions is less than 10 percent.

Willemse found that the skin threshold concentrations for house dust, house dust mite, and human dandruff were the same in the

TABLE 4–7. Pollens of Importance—Area 7

West Kansas, West Oklahoma, West Texas, Colorado, New Mexico, Arizona, Utah		
GRASSES	**TREES/SHRUBS**	**WEEDS**
Bermuda	Ash, Green	Careless Weed
Blue, Kentucky	Ash, Arizona	Cocklebur
Brome	Aspen	Dock, Yellow
Canary, Reed	Box Elder	Iodine Bush
Fescue, Meadow	Cedar, Salt	Kochia
Grama	Cedar, Mountain	Lamb's Quarter
Johnson	Cedar, Rocky Mountain	Marsh Elder
Orchard	Cottonwood, Common	Marsh Elder, Burweed
Quack	Cottonwood, Fremont	Pigweed, Rough
Red Top	Cypress, Arizona	Plantain, English
Rye, Perennial	Elm, American	Povertyweed
Rye, Italian	Elm, Chinese	Ragweed, False
Timothy	Juniper, Pinchot	Ragweed, Giant
Western Wheat	Juniper, Oneseed	Ragweed, Short
Wild rye	Juniper, Utah	Ragweed, Western
	Mesquite	Russian Thistle
	Mulberry, White	Sagebrush, Common
	Mulberry, Red	Sagebrush, Pasture
	Mulberry, Paper	Sagebrush, White
	Oak, Virginia Live	Saltbrush, Annual
	Oak, Gambel	Scale, All
	Olive	Scale, Lens
	Pecan	Scale, Wing
	Sycamore, American	Sheepfat
	Walnut, Arizona	Sorrel, Sheep
		Water Hemp, Western

dog as they were in humans. For animal danders, pollen mixtures, and fungi, he found that the threshold concentration for the dog was ten times higher than it was in humans. For pollens, he found that a concentration of 1000 Noon units/ml was ideal for testing dogs. This is approximately equivalent to 500 PNU/ml. His data do not directly correlate with those in the American literature, since his source of allergens is not available in the United States.

August tested 90 normal dogs with various concentrations of allergens and found an acceptable threshold concentration of 1500 PNU/ml for ragweed, cocklebur, cotton linters, nylon, kapok, pyrethrum, and various mixtures. For house dust, a mold mixture, and a household insect mixture, he found that a concentration of 250 PNU/ml was too irritating. This shows how the irritability of allergens can vary considerably.

Most veterinary dermatologists find that a concentration of 1000 PNU/ml is satisfactory for most allergens. House dust and house dust mite extracts are known irritants and should be used at a

TABLE 4–8. Pollens of Importance—Area 8

Washington, Oregon, Idaho		
GRASSES	**TREES/SHRUBS**	**WEEDS**
Bermuda	Alder, Red	Cocklebur
Blue, Kentucky	Alder, White	Marsh Elder, Burweed
Brome	Ash, Oregon	Dock, Yellow
Canary, Reed	Aspen	Kochia
Fescue, Meadow	Birch	Lamb's Quarter
Oat	Box Elder	Mugwort
Orchard	Cedar, Rocky Mountain	Nettle
Quack	Cottonwood, Black	Pigweed, Rough
Red Top	Elm, American	Plantain, English
Rye, Perennial	Elm, Chinese	Povertyweed
Rye, Italian	Hazelnut Species	Ragweed, False
Salt	Juniper, Utah	Ragweed, Giant
Sweet Vernal	Juniper, Western	Ragweed, Western
Timothy	Maple, Coast	Russian Thistle
Velvet	Oak, Garry	Sagebrush, Mugwort
Western Wheat	Oak, California Black	Sagebrush, Common
Wild rye	Pine, Western Yellow	Sagebrush, White
	Pine, White	Scale, Wing
	Walnut, Black	Sheepfat
	Walnut, English	Sorrel, Sheep
	Willow	

strength of 250 PNU/ml or less. Other questionably irritating allergens are *Rhizopus nigricans*, sheep's wool, silk, animal danders, and mixed feathers. For these antigens, a strength of 500 PNU/ml has been suggested by some authors.

Initially, all allergens except house dust and house dust mite should be used at 1000 PNU/ml, and some normal dogs should be tested. If the reactivity for any one allergen is 10 percent or greater, the concentration should be decreased. Ideally, each new batch of allergens should be tested on normal dogs to make sure that the new antigens are not irritating. Usually this is impossible and is not necessary if the allergens are purchased from the same reputable laboratory. Again, allergy test results should be tabulated, and an indication should be made when a new batch of allergens is used. If there is a sudden increase or decrease in reactivity of a specific allergen, that allergen should be checked for concentration, dating, contamination, and so forth.

Stability of Test Antigens

Allergens are biologic products that lose potency with time. Outdated extracts should be discarded. Loss of potency is affected by the nature of the preservative used, the concentration of the

TABLE 4–9. Pollens of Importance—Area 9

Northern California, Nevada (except extreme southern portion)		
GRASSES	**TREES/SHRUBS**	**WEEDS**
Bermuda	Alder, White	Cocklebur
Blue, Kentucky	Ash, Oregon	Dock, Yellow
Brome	Birch	Greasewood
Canary, Reed	Box Elder	Iodine Bush
Fescue, Meadow	Cedar, Rocky Mountain	Kochia
Johnson	Cedar, Salt	Lamb's Quarter
Oat	Cottonwood, Black	Mugwort
Orchard	Cottonwood, Fremont	Pigweed, Rough
Quack	Elm, American	Plantain, English
Red Top	Elm, Chinese	Povertyweed
Rye, Perennial	Elm, Siberian	Ragweed, False
Rye, Italian	Hazelnut	Ragweed, Western
Salt	Juniper, Western	Russian Thistle
Sweet Vernal	Juniper, California	Sagebrush, White
Timothy	Maple, Coast	Sagebrush, Common
Velvet	Oak, Coast Live	Scale, Lens
Western Wheat	Oak, California Black	Scale, Wing
Wild rye	Oak, California Scrub	Sheepfat
	Pine, Western Yellow	Sorrel, Sheep
	Pine, White	
	Walnut, Black	
	Walnut, Southern California Black	
	Walnut, English	
	Willow	

allergenic solution, the temperature, and the time. Glycerinated extracts tend to lose potency less rapidly but are not satisfactory for intradermal skin testing.

As was discussed previously, phenol-preserved allergens can lose potency rapidly. Allergens kept at 35° C will lose approximately one-half their antigenic activity within seven days. To minimize the temperature-dependent loss of potency, allergens, especially those at skin test strength, should be kept refrigerated. When the allergens are removed from the refrigerator for use, they should be kept cool with refrigerator packs available from the supplier.

One author (LMR) tested 20 dogs with two sets of antigens to determine what effect storage time had on skin test reactivity. One set was freshly made, while the other was constantly refrigerated for 30 days. A correlation of only 20 percent was seen. In those patients in whom the fresh and dated allergens gave dissimilar results, the dated extracts gave false-negative results in 40 percent. Equally interesting was the false-positive rate of 40 percent with the dated extracts. It would appear that stored antigens not only can lose potency but also can undergo degradation that can make them

TABLE 4–10. Pollens of Importance—Area 10

Southern California, Extreme Southern Nevada		
GRASSES	**TREES/SHRUBS**	**WEEDS**
Bermuda	Acacia	Careless Weed
Blue, Kentucky	Ash, Arizona	Burrobush
Brome	Birch	Cocklebur
Fescue, Meadow	Box Elder	Dock, Yellow
Johnson	Cottonwood, Black	Iodine Bush
Oat	Cottonwood, Fremont	Kochia
Orchard	Cypress, Arizona	Lamb's Quarter
Red Top	Elm, American	Pigweed, Rough
Rye, Perennial	Elm, Chinese	Plaintain, English
Rye, Italian	Elm, Siberian	Povertyweed
Timothy	Eucalyptus	Ragweed, Desert
Velvet	Maple, Coast	Ragweed, False
Wild rye	Mesquite	Ragweed, Western
	Mulberry, White	Russian Thistle
	Mulberry, Paper	Sagebrush, Coast
	Oak, California Scrub	Sagebrush, Common
	Oak, Coast Live	Scale, Lens
	Oak, Valley	Scale, All
	Olive	Scale, Wing
	Pine, Australian	Sorrel, Sheep
	Pine, Western Yellow	
	Sycamore, Western	
	Walnut, Black	
	Walnut, Southern California Black	

irritating. Further studies are under way to confirm or negate these findings. Until these studies are completed, the authors suggest that skin test dilutions be replaced every one or two months.

FACTORS AFFECTING SKIN TESTING

Technique, allergen preparation, drugs, inherent host factors, and the season of the year all can affect skin test results and cause false-positive or false-negative reactions. The most common reason for questionable test results is drug interference. Anti-inflammatory or immunosuppressive drugs decrease the reactivity of the skin and interfere with the interpretation of skin test results. Positive results obtained in the face of drug therapy are valid, while negative results are open to question.

Diphenhydramine can suppress skin testing for 1.9 days, chlorpheniramine for 2.5 days, and hydroxyzine for 4.3 days. The authors suggest that all antihistamines be withdrawn at least 7 to 10 days prior to skin testing. In humans, glucocorticoids are not believed to

TABLE 4–11. Skin Test Antigens—Dr. Reedy

GRASSES	WEEDS	MISCELLANEOUS
Johnson	Ragweed	House Dust
Bermuda	Cocklebur	Mixed Feathers
Rye	Marsh Elder	Cat Epithelium
Blue, Kentucky	Careless Weed	Dog Epithelium
Orchard	Sage	Flea
Timothy	Kochia	
Bahia	Russian Thistle	
Quack	Yellow Dock	
	Lamb's Quarter	
	English Plaintain	

TREES/SHRUBS	MOLDS
Mountain Cedar	*Alternaria*
Elm	*Hormodendrum*
Mesquite	*Penicillium*
Oak	*Aspergillus*
Box Elder	

interfere with allergy testing, but this is not so in the dog. The duration of the blocking effect of steroids varies and depends on inherent host factors, the drug used, the dosage, the route, the frequency of administration, and, most importantly, the duration of treatment. Since steroids are absorbed from topical preparations, even otic medications, all routes of administration must be considered. Patients that have been given oral glucocorticoids intermittently, or for two weeks or less, typically can be skin-tested after withdrawal of the drug for two weeks. When injectable drugs have been given, the withdrawal period is longer and is at least four weeks and, more typically, six to eight weeks. Three weeks is suggested as the minimum withdrawal time for dogs who have received chronic steroid therapy, but it can take much longer. The authors have seen patients in which a valid skin test could not be obtained for at least two months after steroid withdrawal. When drug interference from steroids or other therapeutic agents may be a problem, the animal should be tested with the positive and negative controls before the complete skin test is started. If the reactivity of the skin is poor, the complete skin test should be postponed for at least two weeks. As was mentioned before, a reaction to the positive control does not guarantee the remaining test's validity.

Inherent host factors also affect skin test results. Schwartzman showed that very young dogs were less reactive than young adult dogs, and Willemse found a significantly lower frequency of test reactions in dogs older than six years. Young dogs could be less reactive because of their short sensitization periods. Decreased reactivity of the skin with advancing age is recognized in humans.

TABLE 4–12. Skin Test Antigens—Dr. Miller

GRASSES	WEEDS	MISCELLANEOUS
Alfalfa	Plaintain, English	House Dust
Blue, Kentucky	Lamb's Quarter	Tobacco
Fescue, Meadow	Pigweed Mix	Kapok
Orchard	Cocklebur	Newsprint
Rye, Perennial	Marsh Elder	Cottonseed
Timothy	Goldenrod	Sheep Wool
Red Top	Ragweed Mix	Mixed Feathers
Sweet Vernal	Dock-Sorrel Mix	Cat Epithelium
	Dandelion	Flea
	Kochia	

TREES/SHRUBS	MOLDS
Ash Mix	*Alternaria*
Birch Mix	*Aspergillus* Mix
Elm Mix	*Epicoccum*
Maple-Box Elder Mix	*Fusarium* Mix
Oak, Eastern Mix	*Curvularia*
Pine, White	*Helminthosporium*
Poplar, White	*Hormodendrum*
Beech, American	*Mucor* Mix
Walnut, Black	*Penicillium* Mix
Sycamore, Eastern	*Pullularia*
Cedar, Red	*Phoma*
Alder, White	*Rhizopus* Mix
Bayberry	*Stemphyllium*
	Botrytis
	Cephalosporium

Willemse's data from dogs support this observation; he offers the explanations of decreased antibody synthesis, alterations in the effector system, or changes in target organ sensitivity or responsiveness. August found a lower reactivity in adult dogs one to four years of age which could not be explained. August also noted an overall reduction in reactivity as the degree of coat pigmentation increased.

Pregnancy, stress, and serious internal diseases can reduce the reactivity of the skin. Healthy dogs who struggle violently during skin testing apparently release enough endogenous glucocorticoids and catecholamines to reduce or completely block skin reactivity. Because sick or pregnant dogs are "stressed," decreased reactivity can be expected in these patients and the skin testing should be postponed.

In humans, maximum skin test reactivity occurs between 1900 and 2300 hours, while the weakest reactivity occurs at 0700 hours. This probably is due to the circadian variation in plasma cortisol levels. It is not known if this occurs in dogs, but seasonal variations in reactivity do occur.

Immunoglobulins—IgE, IgG_d, or both—are involved in the pathogenesis of atopy. Both have serum and tissue half-lives. When allergen exposure stops, antibody synthesis should stop, and the antibody levels should decrease. Halliwell reported that the radioallergosorbent test (RAST) reactivity of one ragweed-allergic dog varied in excess of 300 percent when samples were taken at different times of the year. As expected, levels in the early summer were much lower than they were during ragweed season. The authors have recognized atopic dogs that failed to react to spring and early summer allergens when the skin tests were done during the winter. Significant reactions were obtained when the test was repeated at the end of the pollen season.

Nesbitt addressed the question of the seasonal variability of skin test results. His data are difficult to interpret, but he found some expected seasonal variations, such as decreased reactivity to grasses during the winter. Unexpected reactions included a decreased reactivity to trees in spring and an increased reactivity to mixed ragweed in the summer before peak ragweed season. The decreased reactivity to trees could be explained by anergy, but the ragweed reaction is hard to explain. Nesbitt proposed that the high allergen load of the summer increases the dog's skin reactivity and, thus, lowers the allergic threshold to allergens. Accordingly, this phenomenon would increase the sensitivity of skin testing or increase the incidence of false-positive reactions.

To minimize confusion and increase the reliability of skin test results, it is advisable to test the animal within 60 days of the end of the allergy season. Tests done before or during the peak pollen period are likely to be unreliable. Tests done prior to the pollen period may be negative (false-negative), because the antibody levels have dropped as a result of no antigenic challenge. Tests done during the peak pollen season can be positive or negative. Negative reactions could be due to drug interference or pollen interference (anergy). During peak pollen periods, the animal can be exposed to such high levels of exogenous pollens that too few sensitized mast cells remain to be detected by skin testing. This anergy decreases as the number of sensitized mast cells increase.

The best time to test an animal depends on the seasonality of its problem. Animals with short, well-defined allergy periods should be tested at the end of the season. Indoor allergic animals will usually react year-round, but the early spring is the best time to test them. During the winter, the indoor allergen load increases because of the closed nature of the house, and animals tend to spend more time inside. When the test is done in the spring, the animal's antibody levels should be at their peak, but the antigen load should be decreasing, so anergy will not be noted.

It is difficult, if not impossible, to define the best time to test a dog with long seasonal allergies, e.g., the dog with perennial allergies or one with allergies from March through December. The authors recommend that these animals be tested in the early winter. At this time, outdoor allergens should be significantly decreased, while indoor allergens should not be high enough to cause anergy. Valid reactions to late summer, fall, and indoor allergens should be obtained, but spring and early summer allergens may be missed. Careful review of the history and skin test results will indicate if the animal's allergens have been well-defined. If the spring and early summer reactions are questionable, the animal should be retested for those allergens in the late spring or early summer. The necessity to conduct several partial allergy tests on an animal with perennial allergies applies to both intradermal and serologic methods of allergy testing.

Some atopic animals will respond well to immunotherapy but will start to scratch again at a later date. A common reason for this is that the animal has become clinically allergic to new allergens. The original skin test results should be reviewed, and the animal should be retested for those allergens that were initially nonreactive.

Skin Test Site and Preparation

By convention, the skin over the lateral thorax is used for skin testing. If the animal is to be tested for only a few antigens, the abdominal skin can be used, but the testing is more difficult. August reported an increased reactivity of the glabrous skin of females.

The site should be clipped carefully with a number 40 blade. If the area is dirty, the site can be gently cleaned with a moist towel, but it should not be scrubbed. Inflamed or infected skin should not be used for testing. If a few pustules or papules are present, the site can be used but these lesions should be avoided.

The skin test sites are marked with a waterproof marker. Typically, a dot is placed on the skin, and the skin above or below the dot is tested. Occasionally, an axonal reflex from a strong positive reaction will enhance the reactivity of adjacent test sites. To avoid this, the test sites should be approximately 4 cm apart.

Skin Test Methods

Direct allergy skin testing can be done by the scratch, prick, or intradermal method. Very minute amounts of allergen are used in the scratch and prick test, and these tests are used in humans to minimize the risk of severe systemic reactions. The prick test is performed by pricking the skin with a needle or lancet and applying a drop of allergen solution. With the scratch test, a scratch is made in the skin, and the allergen is gently rubbed into the wound. With both methods, the patient must remain still for 15 minutes to prevent the mixing of the antigens. The scratch and prick tests are rarely used in animals, since they rarely develop serious reactions to skin tests. Animals also have less sensitive skin than humans and will usually not remain still for 15 minutes.

Intradermal, or more correctly intracutaneous, allergy testing is the method employed in veterinary medicine. Major advantages to this type of testing are that it is more sensitive, more accurate, and easier for the patient than the prick or scratch test. Since this method involves a larger allergenic challenge, false-positive reactions can occur and anaphylactic reactions, although very rare, have been reported.

Technique

Most animals will tolerate a short skin test without chemical restraint. Animals that struggle excessively can become dangerous and may invalidate the skin test because of endogenous steroid and epinephrine release. Vicious animals or those that are expected to resent skin testing should be sedated or anesthetized. Potent hypotensive agents or acepromazine should not be used. In the dog, xylazine (Rompun) or Innovar Vet does not seem to block skin test reactivity; ketamine (Vetalar) is satisfactory for cats. Gas anesthesia can be used in either species. The animal usually is held or placed in a recumbent position for testing.

Most veterinary dermatologists refrigerate their allergens in tuberculin syringes with 26- or 27-gauge intradermal needles. The needles are not changed between patients, unless a needle becomes contaminated, bent, or dull. Needles should be replaced before the syringes are refilled so that the stock bottles will not be contaminated. Since cats are more difficult to test than dogs, the needles should be replaced for cats. Some animals struggle more when the allergens are cold. Allowing the antigens to warm to room temperature decreases the struggling and will not affect potency if the syringes are refilled every two to four weeks. All air bubbles should be expelled before testing. If air is injected with the allergen, a "splash" reaction will occur, reducing the precision and reliability of that test site.

After the test site is marked, the testing can be started. The skin at each test site should be held taut, and the point of the needle is gently inserted in a forward lifting motion, as if to pick up the skin with the tip of the needle. As the tip enters the skin, the pickup motion gradually is converted into a forward and downward pressure, while the syringe barrel is lowered toward the skin. The bevel should lie completely within the epidermis and between the layers of the skin. After the needle is placed, 0.02 to 0.05 ml of the allergen is forced into the skin to form a small bleb. Most clinicians use 0.05 ml as this is easier to measure on the syringe. The volume of test

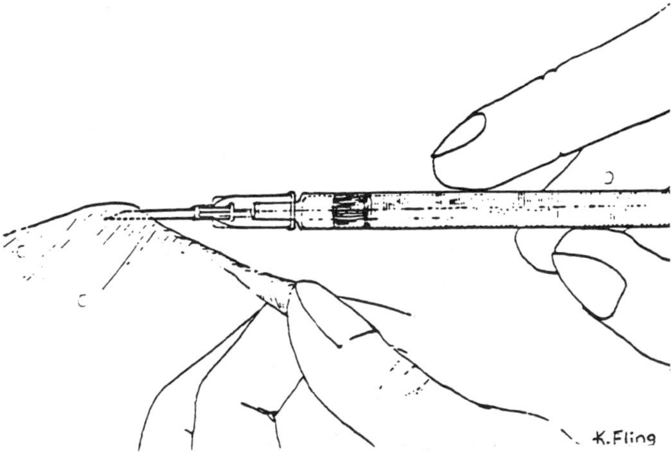

FIGURE 4–2. Schematic of needle placement during intradermal testing.

antigen should be exactly the same at each test site. Figures 4–2 and 4–3 demonstrate the testing procedure.

If the needle is placed too deeply, the normal translucent bleb will not be seen. Hemorrhage also indicates poor needle placement. If a splash reaction occurs or if the needle is placed too deeply, the

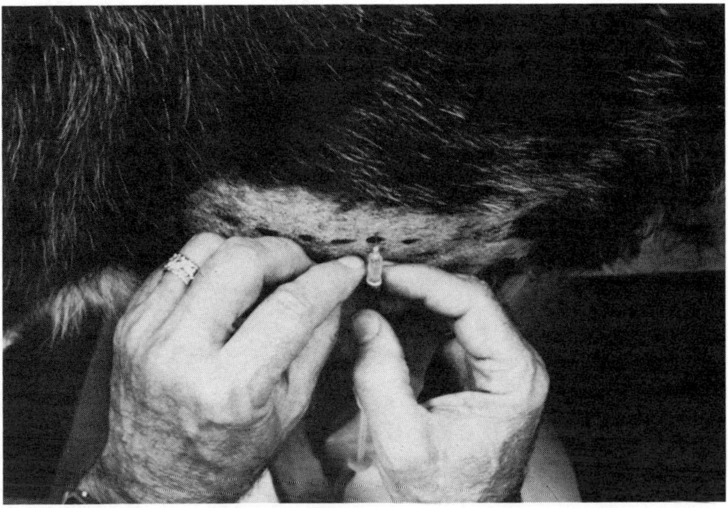

FIGURE 4–3. Intradermal skin testing.

test should be repeated at a new site. Repeating the injection at the same test site can increase the incidence of false-positive reactions at that site and adjacent sites due to an axonal reflex.

After the testing is completed, the anesthesia can be stopped. Manually restrained dogs are allowed to sit up but must be prevented from scratching or licking the test site. Trauma to the test area will make reading the test difficult and can increase the incidence of false-positive reactions.

INTERPRETATION OF SKIN TEST RESULTS

The allergic skin test reaction is a wheal that reaches maximum size 12 to 17 minutes after the injection. The size of the reaction depends on the volume injected, the sensitivity of the mast cell system, and the sensitivity of the patient. Tests should be read 15 minutes after the injections are completed. If a large number of allergens are used, the testing will take at least 15 minutes, and the early injections will be ready to read at the end of the testing. In this case, the test should be read at 15 and 30 minutes to make sure that no significant reactions are overlooked. Cats' skin tests are difficult to read and should be checked at 10, 15, and 30 minutes.

Wheal size and quality are used to grade skin test reactions. The room should be darkened and the test site should be transilluminated with a bright light. This allows better visualization of the size and redness of the wheal. Each wheal should be touched lightly to estimate its turgor.

Positive reactions can be defined by several different methods, each of which has its own advantages and disadvantages. If one is only interested in defining positive and negative reactions, any wheal that is significantly larger (3 mm or greater) in diameter than the size of the negative control would indicate a positive reaction. Simply defining positivity or negativity makes the interpretation of false-positive reactions difficult and places the clinician at a potential disadvantage when antigens are selected for immunotherapy.

Most veterinary dermatologists use a grading system to classify the skin test reactions. Both objective and subjective considerations are included. Wheal size is evaluated objectively. A wheal the same size as the negative control is graded as a 0, while a wheal the size of the histamine rection is a +4. Occasionally, a reaction larger than a +4 will be seen. A +1, +2, or +3 reaction is one that is one-quarter, one-half, or three-quarters the size of the negative and positive control. With experience, this gradation can be determined visually; or the wheal diameters can be measured and the calculations made more precisely.

A permanent record of the skin test can be made as follows. Each wheal is circled with a dark marker; then the row is covered with clear transfer tape (such as Transpore—3M). As the tape is peeled from the animal's body, the marks around the wheals are lifted onto the tape. The tape is then transferred to the medical record, and the wheal diameters can be measured accurately. Since reactions usually are oval or irregular (Fig. 4–4), the average diameter is calculated by taking the sum of the greatest and smallest diameters and dividing by two.

Subjective considerations include the induration, erythema, and the steepness of the wall of the wheal. Flaring and pseudopods, common in human skin tests, are rare in the dog. If two wheals were of identical size, but one was more erythematous and indurated, it would be considered more reactive. Nesbitt estimated that subjective considerations increase the incidence of positive reactions by 20 to 30 percent. A skin test is shown in Figure 4–5.

After the results of the skin test are recorded, the significance of the reactions—either positive or negative—must be evaluated in light of the patient's exposure and clinical history. False-positive and false-negative reactions do occur. Positive reactions can be real or false-positive; true reactions indicate only that the patient has a skin sensitivity. The clinical significance of each reaction is based on the historic correlation.

False-Positive Reactions

Any positive reaction that occurs without a known history of exposure should be viewed as false-positive. Reactions that can be

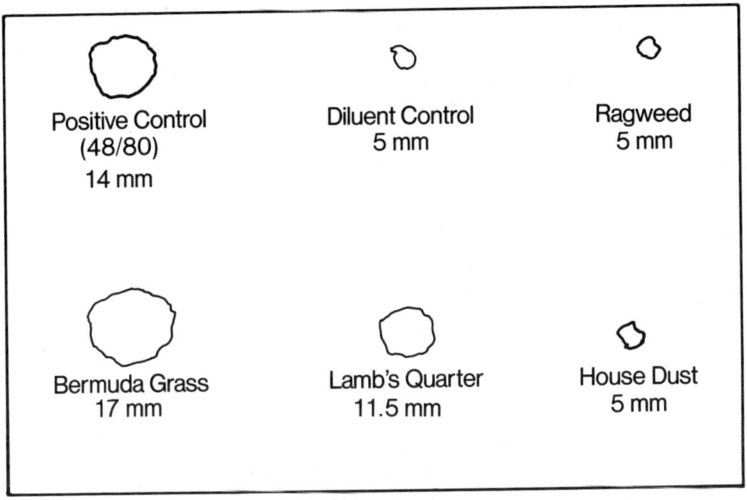

FIGURE 4–4. Outline of allergy test reactions.

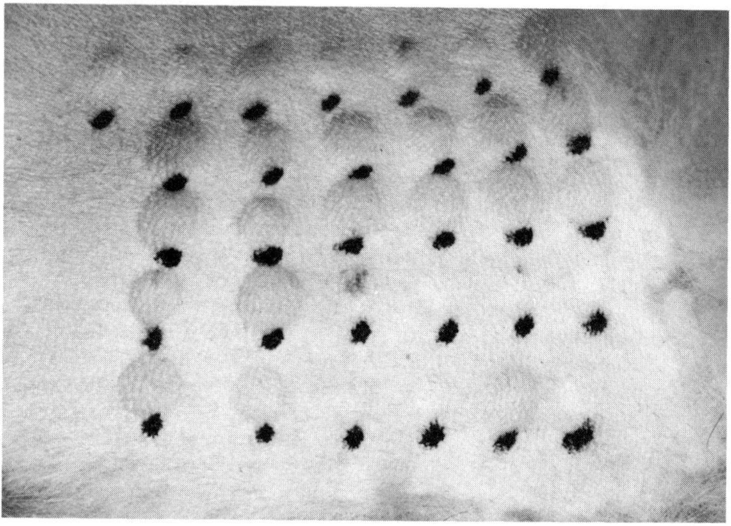

FIGURE 4–5. An intradermal skin test showing many strong reactions.

correlated with exposure but do not fit the animal's clinical history can be insignificant true reactions or false-positive ones. A house dust skin test sensitivity in a summertime pruritic dog could be a true or a false-positive reaction. A true reaction could be the harbinger of a future sensitivity or a remnant of a previous one. A false-positive reaction is obviously of no significance to the animal, but it is important to the clinician.

The common reasons for the occurrence of false-positive reactions are shown in Table 4–13. The most common reason is too concentrated an allergen. Skin test reactions from all skin-tested dogs

TABLE 4–13. Reasons for False-Positive Reactions

1. Improper technique
   - Poor test site selection
   - Poor test site preparation
   - Injections too close together
   - Excessive volume
   - Traumatic needle placement
2. Irritant test allergens
   - Excessive concentration
   - Contamination
   - Preserved with glycerin
3. Irritable skin
   - Injections too close together
   - Dermatographism

should be kept in tabular form, and reactions that do not fit the exposure or clinical history should be identified. If an allergen is causing apparently false-positive reactions in over 10 percent of the test population, the preparation of the allergen should be checked. House dust, house dust mite, sheep wool, and silk are known irritants and should be used at lower concentrations. Epidermals (human, cat, horse), mold mixes, *Rhizopus nigricans,* insect mixes, red ant, tobacco, kapok, mixed feathers, and newsprint also have been reported to cause false-positive reactions. Dogs who are skin tested repeatedly can develop skin sensitivities that are probably not of clinical significance. Reactions in these animals must be evaluated critically.

Dogs with very irritable skin (dermatographism or traumatized skin test site) will often show many positive reactions. If the negative control reaction approaches the size of the positive control reaction, or if the dog shows many positive reactions to allergens which do not correlate with the exposure history, the results of the entire skin test are suspect, and the test should be repeated at a later date.

False-Negative Reactions

False-negative skin test results are frustrating and difficult to evaluate. Common reasons for false-negative reactions are shown in Table 4–14. Not all dogs with classic atopy will react to a skin test. Vollset found that only 65.6 percent of his atopic patients reacted to one or more test antigens, while Willemse and Scott reported frequencies of 81.7 and 90.0 percent, respectively.

The more common causes for a completely negative skin test are that the tentative diagnosis of atopy was incorrect and/or that there was drug interference. If the positive control reaction is not adequate, the test results are invalid. When drug interference is suspected, the patient should be tested with the positive and negative control weekly or bi-monthly until satisfactory reactions occur. Unfortunately, a positive histamine reaction does not guarantee that the skin test will be valid. The histamine reaction tests the reactivity of the skin and not the reactivity of the IgE/mast cell system, which can be less reactive than the skin. If the patient is a strong atopic suspect but does not react to any test antigens, the skin test should be repeated in two to four weeks.

Failure to include the appropriate allergens in the test set also can cause false-negative allergy tests. Most patients presented for skin testing are nonseasonally pruritic, and most skin test–positive dogs react to multiple antigens. If the test antigens are carefully selected, the atopic dog should show at least one reaction.

A more troublesome problem occurs when there are some positive and some negative reactions. The positive reactions indicate that the dog can be tested, but the negative reactions can be true- or false-

TABLE 4–14. Reasons for False-Negative Reactions

1. Improper technique
   - Wrong test site
   - Insufficient volume
   - Injection of air
   - Subcutaneous injection
2. Insufficient allergenic principle
   - Poorly manufactured allergen
   - Old or outdated extract
   - Solution too diluted
     - Mixed antigen used
     - Poorly prepared antigen
3. Drug interference
   - Glucocorticoids
   - Antihistamines
   - Nonsteroidal anti-inflammatory drugs
   - Immunosuppressive drugs
   - Tranquilizers, sedatives
   - Adrenergic compounds
   - Progestational compounds
   - Allergy immunotherapy
4. Inherent host factors
   - Coat pigmentation
   - Stress
   - Estrus, pregnancy, or pseudocyesis
   - Patient's age
6. Incorrect antigen selection
7. Test done at the wrong time

negatives. The historic correlation is very important to differentiate these two alternatives. If the dog is symptomatic during a certain period, but the reactions to the relevant allergens are negative, the reactions may be false-negative. The antigen selection should be reviewed, and the skin test for the relevant allergens should be repeated. If the perennially pruritic dog shows no variation in the intensity of its pruritus, it can be difficult if not impossible to detect false-negative reactions.

OTHER METHODS OF ALLERGY TESTING

A wide variety of laboratory methods is available to assess allergic sensitivity, but these are practical only on a research basis. In clinical veterinary allergy, provocative exposure testing and serologic allergy testing can be used to try to document an animal's sensitivity to a substance.

Provocative Testing

The basis of the provocative test is the purposeful exposure of an animal to a known or suspect allergen. In the clinical situation, a large dose of the allergen is given so serious adverse reactions could occur. Provocative exposure testing is more applicable in food or contact sensitivity, but can be used in other allergic conditions.

To obtain the most meaningful data, the test substance should be as pure as possible. The animal should be allowed to inhale, ingest, or contact the substance for a sufficient period of time to see the allergic reaction. If the animal reacts to a substance, it should be withdrawn, and the animal should be given a sufficient period of time to return to normal before additional testing is done.

In atopy, provocative exposure testing has limited applicability. The test is used to determine the significance of some skin or serologic test results. Since pollens and mold spores are not easily obtainable, provocative exposure testing typically is restricted to indoor allergens. For example, a dog reacts to feathers on the skin test, but the significance of this reaction is uncertain. The animal should be confined to a small, clean room (such as a bathroom), and feathered products from the house should be put in the room. Shaking the objects would increase the concentration of "allergen" in the room and should hasten the animal's response. If the animal is allergic to the objects, the signs should intensify almost immediately.

Aside from the difficulty in obtaining test antigens, provocative exposure testing for inhaled allergens is messy, and the results can be unreliable. Most animals are not accustomed to being confined in the bathroom, and this can cause the animal to become mildly to markedly apprehensive. Very nervous animals may not scratch, even if they are allergic to the substance, so negative results can be inconclusive. Positive results probably indicate a sensitivity, but the reaction may not be as specific as desired. Old feathered products contain feathers, danders, dust, and house dust mites, so the animal could be reacting to one or more of these allergens.

Serologic Tests

Serologic tests are used to measure or estimate the amount of allergen-specific antibody in a patient's serum. In veterinary medicine, two different methods are used commercially. The radioallergosorbent test (RAST) uses radioactively labeled antisera, while the enzyme-linked immunosorbent assay (ELISA) uses antibodies coupled to enzymes.

Both tests are mechanistically very similar. The patient's serum is added to different test wells, each of which contains a different antigen. After an appropriate incubation period, the patient's serum is withdrawn and the test well is washed many times to remove any residual traces of the patient's serum. Next, radioactive or enzyme-linked anti-immunoglobulin antisera is added to the wells and allowed to incubate. After incubation, the wells are washed again to remove any unbound anti-immunoglobulin antisera. In the RAST, the radioactivity of each well is then measured. In the ELISA test, chemicals are added to the wells to cause a color change that can be visualized or measured. The higher the radioactivity count or the more intense the color change, the higher the concentration of anti-immunoglobulin in the well. Since the anti-immunoglobulin binds only to immunoglobulins, the radioactivity or intensity of the color change correlates with the concentration of allergen-specific antibody in the patient's serum.

Species-specific anti-immunoglobuin antisera must be used. To date, these tests are available only for dogs. On a per antigen basis, serologic tests are more expensive than intradermal tests. To minimize the cost of these serologic tests, antigen groups rather than individual allergens are evaluated. Different allergens from similar groups are mixed in one well. Grasses are mixed with grasses, weeds are mixed with weeds, and so forth. The number of wells or groups tested, as well as the number of allergens per group, is variable.

In the original investigatory work on RAST results in dogs, Halliwell found extreme variability in test results depending on which allergen was used. For ragweed, there was an 82 percent agreement between positive skin results and positive RAST results. The positive correlation for house dust mite was 42 percent; for timothy grass, 64 percent; for English plantain, 39 percent; for lamb's quarter, 27 percent; and for dandelion, 12.5 percent. There was no consistent tendency for dogs with stronger skin test reactions to give higher RAST values. He found excellent correlation (100 percent) between negative RAST and negative skin test results.

Utilizing an ELISA method, Willemse found measurable allergen-specific antibody levels in 89 percent of his skin test–positive allergic dogs. Fifty-five percent of his skin test–negative but clinically allergic dogs had elevated titers. Similar to Halliwell, Willemse found that the correlation between skin test and ELISA test results varied with the test antigen. The percent agreement between positive skin test and positive ELISA test results was as follows: house dust, 27 percent; grasses, 17 percent; human dander, 16 percent; spring trees, 7 percent; summer weeds, 7 percent; summer trees, 6 percent; dog dander, 5 percent; and cat dander, 1 percent. The percent agreement between negative skin test and negative ELISA test results was as follows: cat dander, 82 percent; dog dander, 72 percent, summer weeds, 71 percent; summer trees, 70 percent; spring trees, 57 percent; house dust, 48 percent; grasses, 38 percent; and human dander, 34 percent.

Unlike Halliwell, Willemse found that some dogs were negative on skin testing but positive on ELISA testing. The figures were 33 percent for grasses, 32 percent for human dander, 28 percent for spring trees, 17 percent for summer trees, 16 percent for dog dander, 15 percent for summer weeds, 11 percent for house dust, and 1 percent for cat dander.

The results of Halliwell and Willemse are not directly comparable since they used different methods, immunoglobulins (IgE and IgG_d, respectively), allergens, and patients. It would appear, however, that serologic allergy tests are more reliable at detecting dogs that would not react to a skin test than they are at detecting skin test–positive dogs. Willemse's finding of skin test–negative but ELISA-positive dogs can be explained in several different ways. These dogs could truly be allergic to the allergens but showed false-negative skin test reactions or, alternatively, the ELISA reactions could be false-positives. The animal's response to immunotherapy would help answer this question, but these data are not available.

Both the RAST and ELISA tests commercially available in the United States measure circulating IgE antibodies and use allergen groups instead of individual antigens for testing. If IgG_d is important in the pathogenesis of canine atopy as Willemse suggests, the measurement of just IgE would cause an increased incidence of false-negative serologic test results. The low sensitivity of Halliwell's IgE RAST would support that contention. Another common problem in both tests is that group allergens are used. Positive reactions can be difficult to evaluate. A group-positive reaction could be due to positive reactions to each component or to a strong reaction to only one antigen. As a result of this, antigen selection for immunotherapy can be difficult. Another problem is that the serologic test can show positive results, while the skin test for the same antigen is negative. These results could indicate a low level of sensitivity on the animal's part, or the reactions could be false-positives. The authors have seen serologic data in which the dogs are supposedly sensitive to allergens to which they had never been exposed. These false-positive reactions could have been due to technical problems encountered during the testing, or they could point out shortcomings of serologic testing.

Assuming that serologic tests are or could be made reliable, they have several advantages. The office testing is quick and painless for the patient, and the veterinarian does not have to invest in biologic materials that could become dated. The cost to the client will be as expensive, if not more so, than a skin test but, since all veterinarians will be able to do the testing, the additional expense associated with a trip to a veterinary dermatologist will be eliminated. Most of the factors that cause false-positive skin test reactions have limited applicability here. In humans, samples can be obtained while the patient is taking anti-inflammatory drugs. The effects of drug therapy on the canine tests are presently unknown. Steroid therapy can decrease antibody levels such that a strong positive reaction may be reduced to a weak reaction. Accordingly, steroids should be withdrawn for two weeks before the testing. It is advisable to withdraw all drug therapy 24 hours before the testing to negate drug interference. The effects of such factors as pregnancy, external and internal parasites, serious metabolic diseases, and so forth have not been studied. Until information is available about the effects of these conditions, allergy testing should be postponed until the animal is healthy.

As discussed before, the timing of allergy testing can affect the results. Halliwell showed that the ragweed-RAST levels in one dog varied by over 300 percent depending on when the sample was taken. Since serologic tests can detect low antibody levels, the timing of sample collection may not be as critical. The authors suggest that early winter is probably the best time to do serologic allergy testing. If the reactions to spring and early summer antigens do not correlate with the history, those tests should be repeated closer to the allergy season.

The number of reports on the reliability of serologic allergy tests in animals is very limited. Shirk reported an excellent correlation between RAST and skin test results in 50 percent of her patients. Twenty-four percent showed moderate correlation, while 26 percent had poor correlation. A company-generated pamphlet on the ELISA test reports an overall correlation rate of 52 percent between ELISA and skin test results. Some antigens had a higher correlation rate, while others were lower. When there are discrepancies between serologic and intradermal results, one must determine which is correct. As skin testing has been used for years, most dermatologists believe this test to be more reliable. The animal's response to immunotherapy can help determine the accuracy of the serologic test results. Immunotherapy based on RAST results was used in 112 dogs, and Shirk reported that 27 percent showed an excellent response to the vaccine. Thirty-nine percent responded moderately, 24 percent responded fairly, and 12 percent showed no response. These data are in line with those reported for skin test–based immunotherapy.

In human medicine, the rates of correlation between RAST and skin test results vary widely depending on the study, method of skin testing, and the allergen investigated. The original report on RAST testing in humans showed a 68 percent correlation between RAST and intradermal test results. The discrepancies were mostly due to weakly positive skin tests combined with negative RAST results. Less sensitive skin test methods, such as the prick or scratch test, give better correlations with RAST results. Weakly positive intradermal reactions could be true- or false-positives. It is generally agreed that there is good correlation between negative RAST results and negative skin test results, so RAST testing is useful in distinguishing between true- and false-positive intradermal test results.

In humans, the rate of correlation between RAST results and provocative challenge testing is better than the rate of correlation with intradermal testing. When RAST results are evaluated in light of the patient's history, coupled with intradermal, provocative testing, or both, a correlation rate of 90 to 95 percent can be achieved. Thus, it would appear that RAST testing can be very useful in identifying clinically significant allergens.

As a result of the uncertain significance of IgG_d in the dog and problems associated with RAST and ELISA testing, serologic allergy testing may never replace intradermal testing. Until there are good published studies documenting the accuracy of serologic allergy testing and immunotherapy, the authors recommend that all atopic suspects be skin-tested. RAST or ELISA testing should be used when intradermal testing is infeasible because of client factors or drug interference. As was true with intradermal testing, the significance of RAST or ELISA tests must be determined by historic correlation.

5 Immunotherapy

INTRODUCTION

The treatment of the atopic patient must be tailored to the needs of both the owner and animal. The three management options available are avoidance, immunotherapy, and symptomatic therapy. Avoidance is the ideal form of therapy because no drugs are needed and the symptoms would be alleviated with the elimination of the allergen. As most atopic animals are sensitive to many allergens and as most environmental antigens are unavoidable, avoidance is rarely possible. At best, avoidance can decrease the animal's exposure, which may relieve its symptoms. Symptomatic therapy or immunotherapy will be necessary to control the remainder of the problem. Immunotherapy is discussed in this chapter; symptomatic therapy will be discussed in Chapter 6.

Specific immunotherapy was introduced in 1911 by Noon and Freeman; they hoped that this therapy would cause desensitization or a complete loss of sensitivity. Although desensitization was not possible, modulation of the clinical response did occur, so the process was termed hyposensitization. Immunotherapy is now the preferred term for hyposensitization. However, in this manual both terms will be used interchangeably.

Immunotherapy attempts to increase the ability of the patient to tolerate exposure to aeroallergens without developing clinical signs. The patient is injected with gradually increasing doses of specific allergens in an attempt to reduce its sensitivity. Although a great deal is known about immunotherapy, the exact mechanism for its clinical effectiveness is not completely understood. Immunotherapy in the field of allergy may be considered as immunosuppression, in which the production of allergen-specific antibody is inhibited.

CANDIDATES FOR IMMUNOTHERAPY

Immunotherapy is not appropriate for every atopic patient. Animals that are allergic for a short period of time each year are best managed via symptomatic therapy. If the signs last three months or less, medical management should be very rewarding. Animals that show signs for three to six months are problematic, while those with signs lasting six months or longer are candidates for immunotherapy.

If symptomatic therapy involves the use of significant levels of glucocorticoids, immunotherapy should be considered even for those animals with short allergy seasons.

The owner's wishes and needs also influence the selection process. In this situation, some owners refuse to use glucocorticoids in their animals. If the animal does not respond to nonsteroidal symptomatic therapy, immunotherapy may be the only other choice. Alternatively, some owners may want symptomatic therapy regardless of the length of the allergy season or the probability of serious side effects with the medication. No owner should be talked into immunotherapy. The owners should make the decision freely based on sound medical advice and on their own desires and capabilities.

Immunotherapy must be given with some regularity, and the animal must be monitored for signs of adverse reactions. People who travel extensively may not be able to comply with the injection schedule. Although neighbors or dog sitters could give the injections, some owners do not want the headache of setting up a complicated allergy schedule. Some owners are squeamish and cannot give injections. Another person can usually be found to give the injections, but this increases the inconvenience and the expense if a veterinarian is involved. The expense of immunotherapy can be significant, especially if frequent veterinary visits are necessary, and the cost can be prohibitive for some owners. Last, the patience and intelligence of the owner must be considered. Some clients are incapable of understanding or following a vaccine schedule, and the authors are aware of instances in which anaphylactic reactions occurred because the owners did not understand what was expected of them. Additionally, one can never be certain that the vaccine is being given frequently enough to be of any benefit. Some owners demand instantaneous results, which immunotherapy cannot provide. Here, symptomatic therapy can be used initially for the immediate results while the immunotherapy is in its lag phase.

Certain animal factors enter into the final decision about the appropriateness of immunotherapy. Although the vaccine administration is minimally painful, there is still some pain associated with it. Very timid animals may resent the injection so much that they become unacceptable pets, and grumpy animals may become vicious. Vaccines are inappropriate for such animals. Although a young dog may be a candidate for immunotherapy, it may not be best to make a vaccine after only one allergy season. Usually, it takes two or more allergy seasons for an animal to become sensitized to the local allergens. Yearly modification of an allergy vaccine increases the expense and confusion of immunotherapy. The animal's age and degree of sensitivity are used by some allergists in their selection of candidates for immunotherapy. Old dogs and those allergic to a large number of allergens will usually respond to immunotherapy. Age and degree of sensitivity alone should not be used to exclude an animal from the process of hyposensitization.

MODE OF ACTION

A variety of immunologic events occurs during immunotherapy, which help to explain its effectiveness. The first change is an increase in the serum levels of allergen-specific IgG. The IgA levels in some patients also become elevated. These increases can be seen after only a few months of therapy. The IgG antibodies are thought to exert a blocking action in the circulation, which may prevent anaphylaxis and which could explain some of the early improvement seen during immunotherapy. The antibody combines with the circulating allergen and forms immune complexes incapable of causing mast cell degranulation. With less free antigen, there will be less coupling with mast cells. The elevated IgA levels could indicate a local trapping of the allergen at the mucous membranes.

The beneficial effects of the elevated IgG antibody levels are variable. In some studies, the rise in blocking antibody levels correlates well with clinical improvement, while poor correlation is observed in other studies. Measurement of allergen-specific IgG levels does not accurately predict how a patient will respond to immunotherapy. IgG levels will eventually plateau despite the continuation of immunotherapy.

The next change seen during the initial phase of immunotherapy is an increase in the levels of both circulating and bound allergen-specific IgE. Because of this, the clinical signs of some patients will worsen. At this point, there is no demonstrable immunologic hyposensitization, but clinical improvement may be seen.

After prolonged, successful immunotherapy, a decrease in allergen-specific IgE can be demonstrated by skin testing and serologic tests. Levels rarely are eliminated entirely, so a state of true desensitization is not reached. In these patients, the normal post-seasonal rise in IgE antibody levels is abolished, suggesting the development of an immunologic tolerance. This modulation of IgE production is thought to be an effect of immunotherapy on the T lymphocyte population, which regulates antibody production. The decrease in allergen-specific IgE is not sufficient alone to account for the clinical improvement seen with immunotherapy. It is unknown whether IgG_d levels are affected by immunotherapy.

Human allergic patients show a wide variety of immunologic idiosyncrasies that can be affected by immunotherapy. Atopic children have an increased number of IgM-bearing B lymphocytes, and untreated adults have a decreased number of T lymphocytes with receptors for IgG. With successful immunotherapy, the populations of these cells return to normal. Allergen-specific T lymphocyte suppressor cells cannot be found in the blood of untreated atopic patients, but they can be found in those treated with immunotherapy. Considering these findings, it would appear that immunotherapy affects the control mechanisms of the immune response and not just IgE production. Additionally, the mast cells of some patients show decreased sensitivity. Degranulation of these cells requires a greater insult, and there may be a reduction in the total number of chemical mediators released.

SELECTION OF ALLERGENS

Immunotherapy is allergen-specific. If a response is seen, it will be to that allergen or to those that cross-react with it, not to all allergens. A patient who is both grass- and ragweed-sensitive may improve during ragweed season with ragweed immunotherapy, but its grass allergies will not be affected. Accordingly, the significant allergens of the patient should be selected. Allergy test results alone should not be used for antigen selection. Some reactions could be false-positive, while others indicate skin sensitivity without clinical significance. The history must always be considered in allergen selection.

However, it is not wise to select allergens for immunotherapy on the sole basis of historic information. The chance of selecting the correct allergens is low. Immunotherapy with an incorrect vaccine should not be helpful, and it may be detrimental. Animals can develop immunologic sensitivity to antigens that are not allergens. It is unclear whether this immunologic reactivity also means clinical allergy.

In the situation in which the allergic animal shows 10 or fewer good strong (+3, +4) skin test reactions, and these reactions correlate with the history, allergen selection is simple. All allergens are selected. A more troublesome situation occurs when some or all of the skin test reactions are weak (+1, +2). If the history correlates with the skin test results, the antigen should be selected regardless of the strength of the reaction.

A more common situation occurs when an animal has unvarying, perennial symptoms and shows a large number of positive reactions in the skin test. Because of the unrelenting nature of the signs, the history cannot be used to determine the significance of most skin test reactions. Obviously, it is not significant if the animal reacts to an environmental allergen to which it is not normally exposed. After any false-positive reactions are eliminated, one is left with a large number of allergens from which to choose. If all of the reactions are equally strong, all of the allergens would appear to be equally important. More typically, one sees variations in the skin test reactions. Some reactions are +4, some are +3, some are +2, and some are +1. A stronger reaction does not necessarily mean that the allergen is more clinically significant. Wheal size can be affected by the degree of sensitivity as well as by the intensity and time of exposure. However, unless the order of significance can be modified by some historic information, the stronger reactions are viewed as the most significant; these allergens are selected first, followed by the less reactive allergens.

Once the list of significant allergens is developed, one must decide how many to include in the vaccine. If the number of allergens is small, usually 10 or less, all of them should be included. When the number is larger, especially much larger, the choice is not as easy. The number selected varies with the method of vaccine preparation and with the clinician. Allergy vaccines can be produced as single-vial mixtures or each allergen can be kept separately.

Clinicians who use immunotherapy protocols with each allergen in its own vial typically restrict the number of allergens to approximately 10. If a larger number is used, the vaccines become very expensive and cumbersome to administer. Most veterinary dermatologists use single-vial mixtures in which many different allergens are all mixed in one vial. The greater the number of allergens included, the lower the concentration of each individual antigen. By convention, most clinicians include a maximum of 10 to 12 allergens per vial. Nesbitt demonstrated that dogs treated with 2 to 10 allergens responded better than dogs treated with 11 to 20 allergens. When only a portion of the animal's allergens are used for immunotherapy, it is hoped that successful immunotherapy to these allergens will take the animal below its allergic threshold. In successfully hyposensitizing 28 dogs, Scott had to limit the allergen selection in 11 dogs, and these dogs responded as well as the dogs that were sensitive to eight or fewer antigens. When large numbers of allergens are to be used, many dermatologists will use multiple vaccines, each containing 10 to 12 allergens. A few clinicians will include all the allergens in one vial, but there are no published reports on the efficacy of this approach.

ROUTES OF ADMINISTRATION

The subcutaneous route of administration is the most common because it is safe and simple. If aqueous extracts are used, the allergens are absorbed from the injection site quickly, so frequent injections must be given. Although intradermal injections have the advantage of slower antigen absorption, the injections are painful, small doses must be given, and the injection is too technically difficult for owners to administer.

Experimental routes of administration include oral, intralymphatic, and through inhalation. Although oral immunotherapy is safe, it is inferior to parenteral administration. Inhalation technically is very difficult, but there are examples whereby inhalation of high concentrations of pollens has been shown to lead to natural hyposensitization. Intralymphatic injections are used in the immunotherapy of cancer. Within limits, the concentration of the antigen that reaches the lymphoid tissue is important in the development of an immune response. Intravenous, intramuscular, subcutaneous, and intradermal injections all lose a portion of the administered dose before it reaches the lymphoid system. Larger doses are administered to compensate for this loss, but larger doses can increase the potential for side effects. Intralymphatic injections result in maximum lymphoid exposure with small doses. This route of administration will probably never be practical for allergy immunotherapy.

VACCINE PREPARATION

As discussed previously, vaccines can be made as single-vial mixtures or as multiple individual vials. Vaccines can be made by the allergy laboratory that supplies the skin test antigens or by the clinician. Regardless of the source, the vaccine should include only those allergens to which the animal is sensitive. Some companies offer various premade single-vial mixtures that include common allergens. For example, one vial may contain house dust, epidermals, cotton, and kapok. If the animal is sensitive to all of those allergens, the vaccine would be fine. More typically, however, the animal is sensitive to only one or two of the antigens. If the premade vaccine is used, the animal will receive a lower concentration of the significant allergens and may become sensitized to the other ingredients.

Allergy vaccines are available as aqueous or alum-precipitated extracts. Alum-precipitated extracts were developed to slow absorption of the allergens, lengthening the interval between injections and decreasing the probability of adverse reactions. These extracts can cause persistent cutaneous nodules or sterile abscesses, and not all allergens are available. Accordingly, these antigens are not used frequently today. Aqueous extracts are preserved with either phenol or glycerin. Phenolization can cause the extracts to lose potency, especially those with weaker dilutions stored at high temperatures. Cats are very sensitive to phenol, so the potential for toxicosis exists. To date, no reports of toxicosis have been noted in the cat. Glycerin-preserved extracts retain their potency better than phenol-preserved extracts but can cause local reactions. Glycerin-preserved extracts cannot be used for skin testing, so they are of limited use.

A variety of purified or modified allergens are being investigated in humans to see if the incidence of adverse reactions can be decreased, while the ease and effectiveness of immunotherapy is increased. These allergens have not been tested in veterinary medicine.

As discussed previously, aqueous allergens for skin testing should be purchased on a PNU/ml basis and not by weight/volume. This also applies to allergy vaccines. All vaccine protocols use a gradually increasing dose schedule, so at least two vials will be necessary. One vial is the full strength allergen, while the second is a 10-fold dilution. If a third vial is used, it is a 100-fold dilution of the full strength allergen.

Aqueous allergens for immunotherapy can be purchased from the allergy laboratory. Typically, the vaccine can be ordered in a 10,000 PNU/ml or 20,000 PNU/ml strength. When a new vaccine is ordered, one vial of 1000 PNU/ml or 2000 PNU/ml strength is also supplied. If a more dilute vial is needed, it will have to be made by the clinician. Most allergy laboratories will limit the number of allergens in one single-vial mixture. Ten to 12 allergens are common limits. Mixtures count as one antigen, so the vaccine may contain more than 12 allergens. To order the vaccine, one simply indicates which allergens are to be included at what strength and volume. Usually, equal volumes of all allergens are added, but if one considers certain allergens to be more significant, a larger volume of those allergens can be ordered.

If a large number of vaccines are needed each year, it is cost-effective to make the vaccines in-house. Other advantages include being able to make stronger vaccines, having them available almost immediately, and being able to control and change the ingredients at any time. The disadvantages are the cost of the allergen inventory and technician time necessary to make the vaccine. The cost and inconvenience of making allergy vaccines are decreased if vaccines are made on a set schedule, for example, on one day each week, rather than on demand.

Most dermatologists use vaccines at a strength of 20,000 PNU/ml. Nesbitt showed that the response to vaccines at 40,000 PNU/ml was not as good as it was with vaccines at 20,000 PNU/ml. One author (LMR) routinely uses vaccines at the 40,000 PNU/ml strength and believes them to be very effective. If allergens are purchased at a 20,000 PNU/ml strength, the vaccine is made by adding the appropriate volume of each allergen to a sterile empty vial. Since allergens lose potency with time, most allergists dispense them in units of 10 to 20 ml, so that the vial is finished within one year.

If the vaccine is to include many antigens, the volume of each allergen is determined by dividing the volume of the vaccine by the number of ingredients. For a 20 ml vaccine with 10 ingredients, 2 ml of each allergen would be added to the sterile vial. If one allergen is thought to be more important, a larger volume of that antigen can be added so that it is at a higher concentration in the final vaccine. Mixed antigens count as one allergen.

Some allergists purchase antigens in 40,000 PNU/ml strengths because of the cost savings. Not all allergens are available in this strength, making vaccine preparation confusing when different strengths are used. Confusion is minimized if the concentrated allergens are diluted down to the strength of the other allergens before vaccines are made. The phenolized sterile diluent must be used for the dilution. The whole vial of the 40,000 PNU/ml antigen should not be diluted at one time. A 10- or 20-ml vial of vaccine-strength antigen should be made, while the remainder of the concentrated allergen is kept at its original strength.

Some allergens such as house dust are available at a maximum concentration of 10,000 PNU/ml. One simply uses them as if they were more concentrated. If the final vaccine volume is an odd amount, sterile diluent can be added to increase the volume. Accordingly, the final strength of the vaccine may not be 20,000 PNU/ml.

Once the maintenance vial (vial #3) is made, the diluted vial or vials are made by ten-fold dilutions of vial #3. One takes 0.4 ml of vial #3 and mixes that with 3.6 ml of sterile diluent to make vial #2. Vial #1 is made by taking 0.4 ml of vial #2 and adding it to 3.6 ml of sterile diluent. All vaccines should be refrigerated.

VACCINE PROTOCOLS

In veterinary medicine, there is no standard schedule for immunotherapy. Although there are four basic protocols, each has been modified by various dermatologists. Most clinicians report similar success rates with these various protocols, so one protocol would not appear to be better than another. What is unknown is whether a dog that failed to respond to one protocol would respond to another. Until data are available indicating the superiority of a protocol, one should select a schedule and become experienced using it for all dogs. Because of the nature of the atopic patient, the schedule will have to be modified for some dogs. Obviously, if the schedule is being changed for almost all patients, then the basic schedule should be reviewed and modified.

All vaccine protocols involve a loading period and a maintenance phase. During the loading period, the amount of allergen that the animal receives is gradually increased over a period of time, until the maintenance level is reached. The maintenance dose is then continued. Typically, the maintenance dose is set, but some clinicians will push the dose to determine what can be maximally tolerated. The maximum tolerated dose is one just below the dose that will cause clinical signs to recur.

With aqueous immunotherapy, two basic schools of thought exist with regard to the frequency of injections during the loading phase. Many clinicians approach this phase leisurely, giving injections once weekly. Others use a more intense approach, giving injections every other day. A very intense approach, called rush hyposensitization, was developed but is rarely used. The more intense schedules were developed to bring the animal to the maintenance level of therapy more quickly.

Leisurely Low-Dose Schedule

Aqueous single-vial mixtures (multiple antigens all in one vial) are used for this schedule. Most dermatologists use a concentration of 20,000 PNU/ml in the maintenance vial, but some use 10,000 PNU/ml, while others use 40,000 PNU/ml.

INJECTION NUMBER	WEEK	VIAL #1 (200 PNU/ml)	VIAL #2 (2000 PNU/ml)	VIAL #3 (20,000 PNU/ml)	TOTAL DOSE (PNU)
1	1	0.1			20
2	2	0.2			40
3	3	0.4			80
4	4	0.8			160
5	5	1.0			200
6	6		0.1		200
7	7		0.2		400
8	8		0.4		800
9	9		0.8		1600
10	10		1.0		2000
11	11			0.1	2000
12	12			0.2	4000
13	13			0.4	8000
14	14			0.8	16,000
15	15			1.0	20,000

This protocol allows the use of large numbers of allergens. If all of the allergens are mixed in one vial, the protocol is followed exactly. If two or more single-vial mixtures are used, there are two options available. The vaccines can all be given on the same day at the same time, or the injection days can be staggered. The leisurely high-dose schedule, discussed next, apparently has no higher incidence of adverse reactions associated with its massive allergen load. Accordingly, the injections here could be given on the same day. If a reaction occurs, one could not be certain whether the total dose was too much or whether the animal could not tolerate one of the vaccines. If the vaccines are given on a staggered basis, a problem with a specific vaccine might be identified. If no problems are seen during induction, the schedules can be merged during the maintenance phase.

Once maintenance is reached, most veterinarians will gradually increase the interval between the injections until the maintenance injection is given once monthly. Injections are given every two weeks, then every three weeks, and finally monthly. Some clinicians will continue with weekly injections until they determine whether or not the animal will respond to the vaccine. Once a response is seen, the interval is then extended.

Leisurely High-Dose Schedule

This schedule originally was developed for use with alum-precipitated allergens but can be used for aqueous antigens.

INJECTION NUMBER	WEEK	VIAL #1 (1000 PNU/ml)	VIAL #2 (10,000 PNU/ml)	TOTAL DOSE (PNU)
1	1	0.1		100
2	2	0.2		200
3	3	0.4		400
4	5	0.8		800
5	8		0.15	1500
6	12		0.20	2000
7	16		0.30	3000
8	20		0.60	6000
9	24		1.00	10,000

With this protocol, each allergen is used at 10,000 PNU/ml and is kept in its own vial. The dose given is the same for each allergen. If 10 allergens are to be used, the animal would receive a total dose of 10 ml (100,000 PNU) at the ninth injection. Maintenance injections are given every four weeks or so. This protocol has the advantage of having a small number of loading injections and of eliminating the need for custom vaccines. One 10-ml vial of each allergen at 10,000 PNU/ml is ordered. If maintenance injections are given monthly, each vial should last approximately 13 months.

The disadvantages are that large volumes must be given at each injection and, unless the allergens are all loaded into one syringe, multiple injections must be given. The mechanics of loading the syringe or syringes can be cumbersome. If five or fewer allergens are to be given, the cost is approximately the same as it would be with the other protocols. As the number of allergens increases, so does the expense. With 10 allergens, it is twice as expensive. This method cannot be used for very large numbers of allergens, since the cost would be prohibitive and one would run the risk of anaphylactic reactions.

Intense Low-Dose Schedule

Aqueous single-vial mixtures are used at a concentration of 20,000 PNU/ml.

INJECTION NUMBER	DAY	VIAL #1 (200 PNU/ml)	VIAL #2 (2000 PNU/ml)	VIAL #3 (20,000 PNU/ml)	TOTAL DOSE (PNU)
1	1	0.1			20
2	3	0.2			40
3	5	0.4			80
4	7	0.8			160
5	9	1.0			200
6	11		0.1		200
7	13		0.2		400
8	15		0.4		800
9	17		0.8		1600
10	19		1.0		2000
11	21			0.1	2000
12	23			0.2	4000
13	25			0.4	8000
14	27			0.8	16,000
15	29			1.0	20,000

Large numbers of allergens can be used with this protocol. If all allergens are mixed in one vial, the schedule is followed exactly. With multiple single-vial mixtures, the injections can be given on the same day or on different days. If different days are to be used, one vaccine can be given on one day and another on the other day. This intense injection schedule can confuse owners and obviously will not work with more than two vials. The authors have found it best to take one vaccine to maintenance before starting the second vaccine. Once maintenance is reached with the second vaccine, the two vaccines can be merged.

Once maintenance is reached, the interval between injections is expanded. An injection is given weekly, then every two weeks, and finally every three weeks. Typically, maintenance injections are given every three weeks, but this may need to be tailored to the individual.

Intense Rush Schedule

This rush schedule was developed to get an animal to maintenance therapy as quickly as possible. Because of the nature of atopic disease in animals, this protocol is rarely used. The times to consider its use are when the allergy season is fast-approaching or when the allergen is life-threatening, such as a stinging insect. The success of immunotherapy in allergy to stinging insects is unproved in veterinary medicine. One of the authors (WHM) has safely administered insect allergens to two dogs, but its value was never proved because the animals were not stung again. The intense low-dose schedule was used in these dogs.

INJECTION NUMBER	HOUR	VIAL #1 (200 PNU/ml)	VIAL #2 (2000 PNU/ml)	VIAL #3 (20,000 PNU/ml)	TOTAL DOSE (PNU)
1	0	0.1			20
2	4	0.2			40
3	8	0.4			80
4	12	0.8			160
5	16		0.1		200
6	20		0.2		400
7	24		0.4		800
8	28		0.8		1600
9	32			0.1	2000
10	36			0.2	4000
11	40			0.4	8000
12	44			0.8	16,000
13	48			1.0	20,000

This intense schedule requires very careful monitoring in the hospital. When this method was used at the University of Pennsylvania, no adverse reactions were seen, but the potential for anaphylaxis exists. At the first sign of any problem, the protocol should be discontinued. This protocol cannot and should not be used for large numbers of allergens. Once maintenance is reached, the vaccine is administered according to the maintenance regimen used for the intense low-dose schedule.

TIMING OF IMMUNOTHERAPY

Allergy vaccines can be given on a co-seasonal, preseasonal, or perennial basis. The co-seasonal approach involves the administration of the vaccine during the allergy season. In the preseasonal method, the injections are started several months before the allergy season and are discontinued at the end of the season. Most dogs do not respond to immunotherapy for at least two months, so the co-seasonal or preseasonal method may not allow a sufficient time for the animal to respond to the vaccine.

Perennial therapy involves the year-round administration of the vaccine. Nesbitt demonstrated that the success rate of immunotherapy was not influenced by when the vaccine was started. In the animal with seasonal allergies, it is best to start the vaccine during the animal's normal season. This should allow a sufficient period of time for the animal to reach maintenance therapy before its allergy season starts. The vaccine can be started at any time with the perennially allergic animal. For such an animal, the intensity of the vaccine protocol should be constant throughout the year. With seasonal allergies, the vaccine frequency can be decreased during normal season but should be increased again one month before the allergy season starts. In many allergic animals, the normal period is so short that vaccine schedule modifications are more trouble than they are worth.

VACCINE ADMINISTRATION

In animals, the incidence of serious adverse reactions to allergy vaccines is very low; therefore, most clinicians have the clients administer the vaccine at home. The first or first few injections should be given in the veterinarian's office to make sure that the owner knows how to give subcutaneous injections. The injection site should not be rubbed after the shot, as this can increase the rate of absorption.

At home, the owner should refrigerate the vaccine. Some animals resent cold injections. If that is the case, the syringe should be loaded and allowed to come to room temperature before the vaccine is given. The vaccine vial should not be warmed to room temperature, as this will decrease the potency of the vaccine. The owner should use a new syringe and needle for ech injection. Disposable tuberculin syringes with short, fine (25- or 26-gauge) needles work best. With multiple single vials, either the allergens can be loaded into one syringe or multiple injections can be given. If the owners are careful not to mix antigens while they are loading a common syringe, this method is best.

The owner should be sent home with a complete list of instructions on vaccine administration and should be told about various problems that could occur. An example of one author's (WHM) handout is included in the appendix at the end of this chapter. If any problems arise, the owners should be told that they must contact the veterinarian before the next injection is given. Serious adverse reactions are usually preceded by obvious but less significant signs. If early warning signs are overlooked, anaphylaxis could occur at the next injection.

The vaccine should be given at a time when the animal can be observed for approximately 30 minutes. The injection does not have to be given at the same time every day. The owner's presence at home is not enough; the animal should be watched. If reactions are not observed during the loading phase, they are not likely to occur during maintenance, and the observation can become more casual. If the owner notes any problems during the first 30 minutes, the observation should be extended to 60 minutes. The vaccine should not be given around the time of a full meal or heavy exercise, and a full meal should not be given from one hour before to one hour after the injection. One author (WHM) has seen three patients in which anaphylactic reactions occurred when the vaccine was given with a meal. However, there was no report of a reaction when no food was given. It is unknown whether the reaction was precipitated by postprandial splanchnic pooling of blood or some other mechanism. Heavy exercise is avoided to minimize blood redistribution.

Administration Problems

After an initial period of squeamishness, most owners have no problem administering a vaccine. An occasional owner will report that the animal squirms or is too active. The owner should be reminded to warm the vaccine first and then distract the dog. When the dog is put on a table, or is taken outside or to a neighbor's, the distraction should allow the owner to administer the shot. A rare dog will become vicious. In this case, the injection should be discontinued or should be given by the veterinarian.

All too frequently, owners will report that the animal did not get the full dose because the needle pulled out or went through the skin. During the loading phase, unless the owner is sure that the animal did not get any of the vaccine, one can assume that the animal received enough, and the schedule is continued. During maintenance, one-half of a dose should be given unless the owner is sure how much of the vaccine the animal received.

Owners often will report that they missed a shot because they forgot or were away. Regardless of which protocol is being used, the owner should convert the veterinarian's schedule to actual calendar days and dates on a big block calendar. This is especially useful with the intense low-dose schedule and with the maintenance phase of all protocols. If the injection was a few days off, the owner should be told to continue with the original schedule. If the vaccine was one to four weeks off, the schedule is followed, but the dates of the subsequent injection need to be adjusted accordingly. If the animal has not received an injection for nine months or more, new vaccines must be made and the protocol restarted at the beginning. The situation in which an animal has not received an injection for one to nine months is less clear. The longer the interval since the last injection, the more care must be exercised upon its reinstitution. The vaccine should be restarted at last phase of loading. The starting dose depends on the lapse period and is as follows:

LAPSE PERIOD (MONTHS)	STARTING DOSE OF VIAL #3
1–3	0.8
3–5	0.4
5–7	0.2
7–9	0.1

Once the starting dose is given, the remainder of the original schedule is followed.

Adverse Reactions

Adverse reactions to allergy vaccines are infrequent and usually will occur during the loading phase of immunotherapy. If no reactions are seen during the loading period but do occur during maintenance therapy, the animal is receiving too much vaccine and a dose adjustment is necessary.

Adverse reactions include local reactions at the injection site, increased pruritus, and systemic signs. Anaphylaxis, shock, and death are obviously very serious problems, but they are very rare and they are usually are preceded by early warning signs. The owner should be told to watch the animal for personality changes (anxiousness), changes in activity (lethargy, hyperactivity), panting, gastrointestinal signs (increased bowel sounds, frequent swallowing, retching, vomiting, diarrhea), changes in urinary habits, and muscular weakness. If any of these signs is seen, the veterinarian must be consulted before any more injections are given. These signs usually are mild and require no therapy, but if they persist for one hour or worsen, the animal should be examined. Anaphylaxis obviously requires immediate medical attention.

The early warning signs are nonspecific; careful review of the history around the time of injection may indicate some other cause for the sign. If no cause is identified, the owner should give the next two or four injections in the veterinarian's office, and the dose should be reduced by one-half. If a reaction occurs, it can be treated immediately. If no signs occur at the office, the owner can return to administering the vaccine at home. A few dogs will show signs at home but not in the veterinarian's office. This can be caused by the owner's or animal's anxiousness. A few owners are so frightened of giving shots that they might imagine reactions. This fright will disappear with time. Some dogs are so nervous in the veterinarian's office that their behavior or the release of endogenous glucocorticoids and epinephrine masks the signs of an allergic reaction. If the owner is calm, reports of reactions at home should be taken seriously.

Pain or local reactions at the injection sites are uncommon and are usually due to poor injection techniques. The technique should be reviewed. Particular attention should be paid to the size of the needle. Large needles can allow some of the vaccine to enter the epidermis and cause an intradermal reaction. Small needles (25- or 26-gauge) should be used, and the injection site should not be rubbed. If a local reaction occurs despite good injection technique, the vaccine is too concentrated or is being given in too large a dose. Local reactions usually subside within 24 hours and do not require treatment. If the reaction persists or bothers the animal, topical steroids with or without systemic medication will help.

Increased pruritus in the animal is a fairly common complaint of owners especially during the loading phase. Initially, few blocking antibodies are present, so the allergens can bind to sensitized mast cells. A gradually increasing dose schedule is used so that the mast cell degranulation that occurs from the vaccine is at a subclinical level. In some animals, a clinical level is achieved. Unless the pruritus is very intense, the owner should continue with the vaccine. If the increase in pruritus is not too significant, no additional therapy is required. Symptomatic therapy can be used. With intense pruritus, the vaccine dose should be decreased and then very gradually increased. Most animals will become less pruritic as the maintenance phase is reached. An animal that shows a continuous increase in its pruritus during the lag and early maintenance phase should have its vaccine checked for accuracy. If the vaccine is correct, the schedule must be changed. Animals that had no problems during the loading phase but that show increased itching associated with maintenance injections may need a dose adjustment.

ONSET OF IMPROVEMENT

The speed with which an animal responds to immunotherapy is very variable. Some clinicians will encourage an owner to continue with the vaccine for two years before it is deemed a failure, although most dogs will respond within the first nine months if they are going to respond. The exact time when the owners will see a response depends on the severity of the disease, the immunocompetence of the animal, and many other factors. Approximately 25 percent of those that respond will improve within the first three months. Fifty percent respond in three to six months; the remaining 25 percent improve between six and twelve months.

Since the animal's response will not be immediate, medications will probably be necessary to control the pruritus. However, if the animal's pruritus is completely controlled with medication, it is impossible to tell if and when the vaccine became effective. The aim of medical therapy should be to control but not eliminate the pruritus. As the immunotherapy starts to take effect, the owner will notice if the animal's pruritus is completely controlled with those drugs. The dose of the medications is then decreased. As the immunotherapy becomes more effective, the dose of the medications is lowered and hopefully eliminated. Shirk reported that dogs that do not receive glucocorticoid steroids seem to do better. Scott's data do not support this observation.

SCHEDULE ADJUSTMENTS

Schedule adjustments are made to account for adverse reactions or for continued pruritus. Before schedules are adjusted, the animal should be examined to determine if there are any other causes for the adverse reactions or continued pruritus. Local reactions at the injection site usually can be corrected by using less concentrated vaccines or a lower dose. When an animal shows anaphylactic signs with the vaccine, one must evaluate the risks versus the benefits of continuing the vaccine. If the atopic disease is so severe that other modes of therapy are inappropriate, the vaccine should be tried again but with extreme caution. Fortunately, anaphylactic reactions are rare.

If the anaphylactic reaction occurred during maintenance, the history should be examined carefully for precipitating factors. The next four injections should be given at the veterinarian's office at a lower dose, and the animal should receive an antihistamine before the injection. The next injection is given one month after the last one. If a reaction occurs, the vaccine should be decreased again by one-half. If a reaction occurs with this second low dose, the vaccine should be abandoned. If no reactions are seen, the vaccine can continue, and the dose can be gradually increased to the maximum tolerated dose. The need for the antihistamine may gradually diminish.

If the anaphylactic reaction occurred during the loading phase, all injections are stopped for one month, and then the schedule is restarted at the beginning. The injections are given at the clinician's office, and pretreatment with antihistamines is advised. If a reaction occurs again, the vaccine should be abandoned. If the vaccine is the only hope for the animal, and if the reactions are severe but not immediately life-threatening, pretreatment with steroids and antihistamines may be of some benefit.

Animals that exhibit low-level systemic signs when the injection is given at home also should be pretreated with antihistamines. If the signs progress, the dose of the vaccine should be monitored carefully. The maximum tolerated dose will probably be lower than that indicated by the schedule.

The most common reason for schedule adjustment is pruritus. Unless the pruritus is intense, no schedule adjustments are made during the loading period, as this increase in pruritus is usually transient. Antihistamines or other anti-inflammatory drugs or both can be used. With intense pruritus, a lower vaccine concentration should be used during the loading phase. Once maintenance is reached, the strength can usually be increased.

During maintenance, some animals will scratch more immediately after the injection, especially with the first injection of a new vial. If the increased pruritus is associated with the use of a new vial, schedule adjustments are usually not necessary. One author (LMR) routinely suggests that the first dose of a new vial be reduced by 50 percent. If the increased itching occurs with an old vial or persists with the new vial, the dose of the vaccine should be decreased until the pruritus stops. In some dogs, this decrease in dosage must be coupled with an increase in the frequency of administration. Some owners will report that the pruritus stops with the injection but returns before the next shot is due. A larger volume of allergen can be given or, more preferably, the frequency of injections can be increased. If the animal's pruritus starts to increase at day 10, for example, the injections should be given every 10 days. If an animal needs a dose adjustment, this will usually happen during its peak allergy season. As the peak passes, the injection frequency can usually be decreased to the original level. If an animal needs a schedule adjustment in one year, it probably will need one in subsequent years.

During maintenance, some owners will report some improvement or no change. Schedule adjustments should not be made before six months as the vaccine may not yet have reached maximum effectiveness. After this time, the dose or frequency or both should be increased to see if improvement occurs. Increasing the frequency to every 10 to 14 days is the preferred method. If the animal improves with this initial schedule adjustment, further refinements in the schedule should be made until the best results are seen. In one case, the dog did not respond until the injections were given every third day. If the animal shows no response to four of these more frequent injections and has been receiving the vaccine for at least nine months, the vaccine is probably of limited or no use.

Flares During Immunotherapy

Some animals that are successfully managed with immunotherapy may experience a flare in their condition. If the signs start suddenly, the animal should be examined especially for fleas or pyoderma or both. Flares owing to inhalant allergens are usually more gradual in onset and can be due to heavy pollen loads or can indicate that the animal has developed new sensitivities. If a schedule adjustment does not help, new sensitivities probably have developed. Immunotherapy is allergen-specific. Successful therapy modulates the immune response to that specific allergen and to any that may cross-react with it—but not to all allergens. When new sensitivities are suspected, the animal should be tested again; new allergens may need to be added to the vaccine, or a new vaccine may need to be started.

RESPONSE TO IMMUNOTHERAPY

In veterinary medicine, response to immunotherapy is often vaguely described as "improvement," and the response rate of dogs ranges from 50 to 100 percent. The definition of success varies greatly, especially when owner expectations are considered. Some owners will expect a complete elimination of signs; others will deem the vaccine successful even though the animal's signs decreased only moderately. Willemse considers immunotherapy successful if his patients improve at least 51 percent, while Scott defines success as the complete elimination of clinical signs. If one couples the problems of terminology with the fact that the various authors use different patients, allergens, extracts (aqueous or alum-precipitated), and schedules, it becomes obvious that it is difficult to draw firm conclusions from the literature.

For the sake of this discussion, the authors would define an excellent response as one in which there is a 75 percent or greater improvement. A good response accounts for 50 to 75 percent improvement, and a poor one allows an improvement of 25 to 50 percent.

From the literature, the average response rate for each category and the range reported is as follows: excellent—36 percent (21 to 60); good—30 percent (21 to 42); fair—19 percent (14 to 24); and poor—22 percent (14 to 35). The ranges obviously are very wide, and some reports are more widely divergent. In one series of 28 dogs, Scott reported the complete elimination of signs in 100 percent of the cases. This figure is unrealistic, and he did comment that a success rate of 60 percent would be more accurate.

To simplify the discussion with owners when they ask the question of what they can expect from immunotherapy, it is best to reduce the number of categories to three—excellent, good, and poor. Excellent and poor are as previously described, while a good response covers the vague ground in between. These categories are very broad and are subject to interpretation by owners and veterinarians. If the owner is very demanding and will accept nothing short of complete resolution of the signs, the failure rate will be much higher.

The failure rate of 22 percent is reasonable, as is the 36 percent response in the excellent category. Overall, one can say that there is a 78 percent response to immunotherapy. If owners are more demanding and require a response of 50 percent or greater, the response rate would be approximately 62 percent.

In a survey of 144 patients on immunotherapy for at least one year, one author (WHM) found that 64 percent of his clients were satisfied with the program, while 36 percent were dissatisfied. In 42 percent of the dogs, immunotherapy was the only therapeutic regimen necessary. Typically, these dogs remained symptom-free as long as the vaccine was given. The other author (LMR) finds that between 75 and 85 percent of his patients will show a good or excellent response.

In one of his papers, Nesbitt observed that younger dogs responded better to immunotherapy than older ones. In a later paper in which he studied a different population of dogs, he found that the age of the patient had no bearing on the success rate of therapy. The data of Willemse, Scott, and the authors support this observation. Nesbitt also observed that the animal's breed was not a factor, but that the females in his population responded better than males. Both he and Willemse do not believe that the number of allergens in the vaccine affects the success rate.

One author (LMR) has made the observation that dogs allergic to pollen respond better (81 percent versus 59 percent) to immunotherapy than those that are not pollen-allergic. Nesbitt reported that dogs with positive reactions to mixed epidermals and grasses responded better than dogs with negative reactions to these allergens. Since most clinicians deal with perennially atopic dogs, these trends are difficult to document. Nesbitt also observed a trend toward a higher rate of success when individual mold, tree, and grass allergens were used. He found equal success using individual and mixed epidermals but greater success with mixed weeds.

In a double-blind study, Willemse found that 21 percent of the dogs in the placebo group improved 51 percent or more and that 80 percent of those dogs became symptom-free by the vaccine. In his double-blind study on immunotherapy for flea allergy, Halliwell found some improvement in the placebo group. Forty percent of the owners felt that there was some change with the placebo, while 20 percent saw a marked improvement. The investigator's grading of the group's improvement was 13 percent. This information points out the need for the veterinarian to assess the dog's response and not to just rely on the owner's observations. Owners can be overly optimistic or pessimistic and make erroneous judgments about the success of immunotherapy.

Because Willemse personally evaluated his patients, it is hard to ignore the observation that 17 percent of the placebo group became asymptomatic. He used alum-precipitated allergens, so his placebo injection included aluminum hydroxide as an adjuvant. Adjuvants stimulate the proliferation of reticuloendothelial cells; therefore, the placebo injections may have modulated the animal's immune response such that they no longer had an allergic tendency or that they underwent spontaneous hyposensitization. If the adjuvant does modulate the immune response in atopic dogs, alum-precipitated vaccines would be preferred. Scott's unprecedented 100 percent cure rate in 28 dogs occurred with the use of alum-precipitated vaccines. Kunkle, however, found that 59 percent of the patients on aqueous immunotherapy improved 50 percent or more compared with only 41 percent of the patients on alum-precipitated programs. All three authors used different immunotherapy schedules, so it is difficult to compare the results. Adjuvant-containing vaccines warrant further evaluation.

As was discussed before, feline atopy is a newly reported disorder, so there are very few reports on the efficacy of immunotherapy in the cat. Scott reported a 100 percent success rate in hyposensitizing three cats with miliary dermatitis. McDougal reported on 13 cats and found that 69 percent improved 75 percent or more with immunotherapy. Three cats improved from 50 to 75 percent; one cat responded poorly. One author (LMR) hyposensitized 15 cats and found that 67 percent improved by at least 75 percent. These data indicate that cats can respond to immunotherapy.

When owners have animals that improve with the immunotherapy, they have a tendency to stay in contact with the veterinarian. If the owner does not notice any change, the temptation is to discontinue the vaccine and return to symptomatic therapy. During the first year of immunotherapy, it is very important to stay in contact with the client at least every two months. If owners do not report in on schedule, they should be called. Animals that are improving are continued on the same therapy. Animals that show little or no response should be brought in for re-evaluation and a possible schedule adjustment. A schedule adjustment will often improve the animal's response but usually will not convert a nonresponder to one that is symptom-free. Although both the client and veterinarian would like a 100 percent success rate, it is not possible with the current state of the art. If immunotherapy significantly reduces the level of medications necessary to control the pruritus, the vaccine should be considered somewhat successful and it should be continued.

Immunotherapy Failures

Between 15 and 25 percent of the patients receiving immunotherapy show little or no response to the vaccine. Unfortunately, if there is no communication with the client, the percentage will increase, since owners often fail to recognize that a significant decrease in medication levels is better for their pet's welfare. Some owners will call immunotherapy a failure if the animal has to take any other medication.

If there is no change with the vaccine after one year of treatment, the immunotherapy should be stopped. Occasionally, a dog will get worse when the vaccine is withdrawn, but most do not. In such a scenario, the immunotherapy should be reinstituted, or the dog should be skin tested again to determine if new allergens can be identified. Many owners will not follow through with this request.

In all cases, the clinician should examine the animal before declaring failure. The authors find that the major causes of apparent immunotherapy failures are secondary infections, fleas, other concurrent allergic disorders (food or contact hypersensitivity), failure to identify or include all pertinent allergens in the vaccine, and the development of new allergies. Few animals require retesting, but those that do usually show an initial improvement with the immunotherapy. As new allergens become significant, there is a resurgence of symptoms that are not due to fleas and the like. Other causes for the failure of immunotherapy include incorrect diagnosis, incorrect vaccine, the animal's inability to respond, and other unknown factors.

Long-Term Immunotherapy

In humans, no adverse effects of long-term immunotherapy have been recognized, and this also appears to be true in dogs. It has been reported that some dogs will be permanently "cured" after one or two years of immunotherapy. This is not the author's experience. Most, if not all, animals will start to show allergic signs without their vaccines.

Appendix A

FACT SHEET FOR VACCINE ADMINISTRATION

Vaccine Handling

1. The vaccine vials should be refrigerated.
2. Vials #1 and #2 should be discarded when the schedule indicates that they are finished.
3. Vial #3 is the maintenance vial. When you are halfway through your last vial, please contact your veterinarian so that more vaccine can be ordered for your animal.

Vaccine Schedule

1. The schedule for administration is attached. Injections are given every other day until day 31. After the injection on day 31, the interval between the injections increases to once a week (day 38), then every two weeks (day 52), and finally every three weeks (day 73.)
2. Most owners find that converting the schedule to actual calendar days and dates is helpful. If a big-blocked calendar is used, the dose can be indicated on the calendar.
3. The schedule is a standard one. Dose adjustments do need to be made for individual patients. Your veterinarian will advise if that is necessary for your animal.

Vaccine Administration

1. The vaccine is given by subcutaneous injections according to the vaccine schedule. Once you have learned how to give the injections, you can administer the vaccine at home.
2. A new needle and syringe should be used for each injection. Carefully save the used syringes and needles and return them to your veterinarian for safe disposal.
3. During the initial phase of the vaccine protocol (day 1 to day 73), the injection should be given when the animal can be observed for 30 to 60 minutes. The injections need not be given at the same time each day.
4. The animal should not receive a major meal one hour before or one hour after the injection. A snack or treat after the injection is allowed.

5. Heavy exercise should be avoided for one hour after the injection. Walks are allowed.
6. If any adverse reactions are seen after an injection, no more injections should be given until you contact your veterinarian. If your animal appears to be seriously ill, you should contact your local veterinarian or veterinary dermatologist immediately.

Adverse Reactions to the Vaccine

1. Adverse reactions are very infrequent. Many animals will become more itchy during the initial phase of the vaccine. If this becomes severe, contact your veterinarian.
2. Aside from an increase in itchiness, adverse reactions are very rare. If an adverse reaction is to occur, there are usually early warning signs. If these early signs are ignored, an adverse reaction may occur. If your animal is not its normal self after an injection, contact your veterinarian. Animals that sleep excessively, are hyperactive, or look uncomfortable after the injection may be showing the first signs of a vaccine reaction. Contact your veterinarian before giving any more injections.
3. Serious reactions are rare, but they can be life-threatening. Labored breathing, vomiting, diarrhea, collapse, or hives over most of the body require immediate veterinary attention. No more vaccine shots are to be given until your veterinarian can review the case.

Points of Information

1. Since the vaccine does not reach "full strength" until day 73, most animals will not show any improvement during the loading phase.
2. Most animals that respond to their vaccine will do so during the first six months of therapy. A few animals will not respond until the end of the first year.
3. Since the vaccine does not work immediately, medications can be used to relieve your animal's itchiness. Your veterinarian will make various suggestions that you should follow. Excessive medication makes it impossible to determine if the vaccine is helping.
4. Routine immunizations should not be given on the same day as an allergy injection. If your animal develops some unrelated medical or surgical problem, contact your veterinarian to see how the vaccine schedule should be modified.
5. If an injection date is missed by up to one week, give the next scheduled injection and follow the schedule. If a longer period of time has elapsed, contact your veterinarian before administering the next injection.

6 Symptomatic Therapy for Allergic Diseases

INTRODUCTION

As discussed throughout this text, avoidance therapy or immunotherapy is most desirable but not always possible. Some owners do not want to or cannot investigate the problem. In other situations such as in the atopic dog with a very short allergy season, immunotherapy is inappropriate. Finally, there are those animals that defy diagnosis or respond incompletely to specific therapy. Symptomatic therapy must be used in such cases.

Symptomatic therapy involves nonspecific agents and anti-inflammatory drugs. The specific protocol depends on the nature of the animal's disease and on the wishes and capabilities of the owner.

NONSPECIFIC AGENTS

Allergic animals have sensitive skin and are prone to bacterial skin infections. Any time an owner reports that an animal with a previously well-controlled condition suddenly starts to scratch, a bacterial or flea problem should be suspected. If a pyoderma is present, antibiotic therapy will usually resolve the infection and return the animal to its previous state. In some allergic dogs, bacterial infections are almost constant. These infections can be a result of an immunologic defect or secondary to the trauma inflicted on the skin when the animal scratches. If an immunologic defect exists, bacterin therapy may be of some benefit (see Chapter 10). If the infections are strictly secondary to the pruritus, more aggressive antipruritic therapy is necessary. In some dogs, the pyoderma will continue to recur. In this case, chronic antibiotic therapy may be necessary.

Fleas obviously are a problem in the hypersensitive animal, but they also can cause a significant problem in those with other forms of allergy. Flea eradication is called for, but the agents used should be selected carefully. Harsh dips and sprays will dry the skin and may cause the allergic dog to itch more. Products containing alcohol should be avoided. Bath oils should be added to flea dips to minimize their drying effect. Pyrethrins are botanic insecticides prepared from the heads of the chrysanthemum plant. Because this chemical can cross-react with ragweed, an atopic dog may be made worse by its use, although the authors have not seen this happen. If the condition of an atopic dog is aggravated by these products, they should be discontinued immediately.

Other nonspecific modes of therapy depend on the distribution and nature of the animal's signs. In those situations in which there is local or generalized pruritus without secondary skin changes, nonspecific therapy will probably be of little benefit. When seborrheic changes occur, antiseborrheic therapy will usually lessen the animal's pruritus. Because allergic dogs have sensitive skin, the mildest antiseborrheic agent should be used. Tar-based products should be avoided. Animals with dry skin should be bathed with Allergroom (Allerderm), HY-LYT efa (DVM), or Nolvasan (Fort Dodge). If the skin remains dry after the bath, bath-oil rinses with Humilac (Allerderm), HY-LYT efa (DVM), or sesame oil (VDP) can be beneficial. Dogs with greasy skin can be bathed with benzoyl peroxide products (OxyDex [DVM], Pyoben [Allerderm]) or sulfur-based products (Sebbafon [Winthrop], SebaLyt [DVM], Sulfur Shampoo [Adams]). If these shampoos are used excessively, they can dry and irritate the skin. Once the greasiness disappears or if irritation is seen, use of the shampoo should be discontinued and a milder one selected.

Focally pruritic animals such as those that scratch their ears or lick their feet may benefit from the application of Domeboro's solution one to three times daily.

These nonspecific modes of therapy at best will decrease the level of pruritus but will not eliminate it. If both the animal and owner are comfortable with the degree of itchiness, no further therapy is necessary. Usually additional therapy is necessary. The aim of medical therapy is to provide the desired results with the least possible side effects. Since many medications are available, it is often a matter of trial and error to find the best drug for each individual patient. Some owners are unwilling to experiment.

ANTI-INFLAMMATORY DRUGS

Allergic diseases are inflammatory disorders, and anti-inflammatory drugs can lessen or eliminate the signs of the disease. There are many anti-inflammatory drugs and more are being developed.

In the treatment of allergic diseases, corticosteroids, antihistamines, and nonsteroidal anti-inflammatory drugs are used most frequently.

Corticosteroids

The cortex of the adrenal gland produces aldosterone, corticosteroids, and the sex steroids. In the dog and cat, cortisol is the primary corticosteroid produced. In the dog, the total daily corticosteroid secretion rate is 1.2 mg/kg, while the cortisol secretion rate is 0.76 mg/kg/day. Corticosteroid production is under the control of the hypothalamic-pituitary-adrenal axis (HPAA). Adrenocorticotropic hormone (ACTH) is released from the pituitary under the influence of blood cortisol levels and other higher influences. ACTH levels and, consequently, cortisol levels are regulated by blood cortisol levels, "stress," and a circadian (diurnal) rhythm.

Cortisol secretion is not constant throughout the day but rather fluctuates according to a circadian rhythm. Both ACTH and cortisol levels are highest in the early morning and gradually decrease during the day. Because of its nocturnal nature, the cat appears to have a reversed rhythm with peak levels occurring during the evening. Stress, which can include fright, cold, exercise, or trauma, can override the circadian rhythm and cause increased levels. Cortisol levels, either endogenous or exogenous, act through a negative feedback loop to alter ACTH and cortisol secretion. Chronic steroid abuse will cause HPAA suppression. Severely suppressed animals will not be able to respond to stress and a shock-like condition can occur.

Adrenal corticosteroids have both glucocorticoid and mineralocorticoid activity. Glucocorticoids were introduced into clinical use in 1949. Modification of the basic steroid molecule has increased the glucocorticoid activity while diminishing the mineralocorticoid effects. The relative potency of the various corticosteroids is shown in Table 6–1.

The physiologic effects of pharmacologic levels of glucocorticoids are caused by the alteration of glucose, protein, and lipid metabolism and by a modulation of the immune response. Steroids modulate inflammation by altering macrophage function (decreased phagocytosis and response to lymphokines), altering lymphocyte function (decreased proliferation and antigen processing), lessening vascular permeability, decreasing release of vasoactive amines, inhibiting prostaglandin and leukotriene synthesis, reducing serum complement levels, redistributing leukocytes, and stabilizing plasma membranes. In general, glucocorticoids have a greater effect on leukocyte traffic than on function. The neutrophilia seen with steroid administration is caused by an accelerated release from the bone marrow, an increase in the circulating half-life of the neutrophil, and a

TABLE 6–1. Relative Potency of Various Corticosteroids

	GLUCO-CORTICOID POTENCY	MINERALO-CORTICOID POTENCY	EQUIVALENT DOSE (MG)
Short-Acting (<12 Hours)			
Hydrocortisone	1.0	+ +	20
Cortisone	0.8	+ +	25
Intermediate-Acting (12–36 Hours)			
Prednisone	3.5	+	5
Prednisolone	4.0	+	5
Methylprednisolone	5.0	0	4
Triamcinolone	5.0	0	4
Long-Acting (>48 Hours)			
Paramethasone	10.0	0	2
Flumethasone	15.0	0	1.5
Betamethasone	25.0	0	0.06
Dexamethasone	30.0	0	0.75

decrease in neutrophil egress from the blood. These changes decrease the number of neutrophils in the inflammatory site and lead to a decrease in inflammation. Steroids themselves do not decrease antibody production. Steroid modulation of cellular interaction can result in a dampening of the humoral response.

The occurrence and severity of side effects observed with steroid administration depend on the drug used, the route, frequency, and duration of administration, and the animal's metabolic status and idiosyncrasies. Cats are resistant to but are not immune from steroid side effects. Steroid side effects can be divided into those that are clinically obvious and those that are biochemical or immunologic in nature.

Clinical side effects always include polydipsia, polyuria, and polyphagia. These signs typically are dose-dependent, although some dogs will show profound signs even with very low doses. In many instances, the severity of these signs is associated with use of prednisone or prednisolone. Usually, switching the animal to an equipotent dose of another steroid that has no mineralocorticoid activity decreases the polydipsia and polyuria to acceptable levels. Weight gain, personality changes, and excessive panting are other common findings.

With more chronic use or increased sensitivity on the animal's part, one sees muscle wasting, weakness, fat redistribution, and dermatologic changes. Skin signs include a poor coat that does not regrow, thin skin, comedones, seborrhea, and increased sensitivity to bacterial infection. Some animals will develop calcinosis cutis. Internal changes include HPAA suppression, eosinopenia, neutrophilia, lymphopenia, hypercholesterolemia, hyperglycemia, elevation of the liver enzymes, and subnormal thyroid function.

Glucocorticoids are not innocuous, and they should be used carefully. Topical products have the widest safety margin, while injectable drugs are the most dangerous. Because of the widespread nature of allergic diseases in animals, topical products cannot usually be the sole mode of therapy. In some instances, judicious use of topical steroids will allow the clinician to lower the dose of oral steroids or to use some other more innocuous anti-inflammatory agent.

Topical Steroids

Because of the hairiness of animals and their habit of licking off topical medications, topical steroids have limited use. Additionally, the use of these products is expensive and requires considerable effort on the owner's part. However, dogs with allergic otitis externa or with focal areas of pruritus may benefit from topical steroids.

In using topical products, one must select the drug as well as its vehicle, as most steroids are available in a cream, ointment, gel, lotion, or spray form. For acute eruptions, the lotion or gel form should be used, while creams and ointments are reserved for chronic lesions. Initially, a potent fluorinated steroid should be used three or four times daily. If the condition is to be managed with topical products, the potency is decreased as healing occurs. Betamethasone valerate and 1 percent hydrocortisone are widely used products. Long-term use of a potent topical steroid can cause local atrophy of the skin, HPAA suppression, and iatrogenic hyperadrenocorticism.

Oral Steroids

The oral route of steroid administration is most preferred because the dosage can be controlled carefully and the drug can be discontinued quickly if necessary. Many veterinarians administer an injection of a steroid, usually of a respositol nature, and follow it with oral medication. This practice should be discouraged, since it increases the cost and potential risk of steroid therapy and usually is no more effective than appropriate oral therapy.

If oral steroids are to be administered for two weeks or less, any drug can be used. Although an occasional dog will show signs of glucocorticoid insufficiency when the therapy is abruptly discontinued, most dogs will not. An anti-inflammatory induction dose of prednisolone is 1.1 mg/kg/day. Classically, prednisolone has been used twice daily, but many dogs will do well with therapy once daily, and this tends to minimize the clinical side effects. If another drug is used, it should be administered at an equivalent dose.

If long-term steroid therapy is necessary, daily therapy is contraindicated. For maintenance therapy, alternate-day therapy should be used, as this minimizes HPAA suppression and steroid side effects. Because of their short half-lives, prednisone, prednisolone, and methylprednisolone should be the only drugs used. After the acute symptoms are resolved, the therapy is switched to the alternate-day regimen and then the dose is decreased to the lowest possible acceptable level. The alternate-day approach is achieved by taking the lowest daily dose that will control the symptoms and increasing it by one-half to three-quarters. This dose is given every other morning and can be adjusted up or down as needed. Some animals may only have to take the medication once or twice weekly.

Again, depending on the situation, steroid therapy should not be the first treatment for atopy but should be used only when other drugs have failed. Even though these other drugs may not be effective by themselves, they still may be of some benefit in lessening the dose of steroids required for maintenance. Once the maintenance level of steroids has been determined, these other drugs are added to the therapy to determine if a reduction in the dose of steroids is possible. Oftentimes antihistamines will lower the maintenance dose of steroids. If antihistamines are not effective, other drugs should be tried. To many owners, this can seem like needless experimentation because the steroids work so well. It should be emphasized to the owner that this experimentation is necessary to determine the lowest possible steroid dose.

When steroids are used for chronic maintenance therapy, the final dose should be one at which the animal is comfortably itchy. If the dog is itch-free, it is receiving too many steroids, and the dose should be reduced. By maintaining the animal at a low level of pruritus, the natural progression or regression of the disease can be followed. In many patients, the maintenance level of the steroid will have to be increased to compensate for the increasing severity of the allergic symptoms. In some animals, one type of steroid, e.g., prednisolone, will seem to lose its effectiveness even at increased dosages. If the animal is treated with an equipotent dose of another steroid, e.g., dexamethasone, the steroid responsiveness can be restored. This apparent resistance to one steroid is called steroid tachyphylaxis, and the phenomenon is poorly understood. After some period of time, the original drug will again become effective.

Dogs receiving chronic steroid therapy should have a complete physical examination at least twice yearly. Since these dogs are prone to urinary tract infections, a urinalysis should be part of each visit. Blood work is run as needed. If there are steroid changes, the therapy can be modified; or, if steroids are the only effective form of therapy, the owner can be informed that changes are occurring and must be followed carefully.

Injectable Steroids

Parenteral glucocorticoids vary in potency, route of administration, and rate of absorption from the injection site. The basic steroid molecule is conjugated to an ester base. Modifications of the ester base change the steroid's water solubility, which alters its rate of absorption. The hemisuccinate or phosphate bases have a very high water solubility with complete absorption in 30 to 60 minutes. The acetate, diacetate, tebutate, acetonide, and hexacetonide bases give poor water solubility with absorption in 2 to 14 days.

Parenteral steroids, even those with the hemisuccinate or phosphate bases, do not have an immediate onset of action. The steroid's mechanism of action is via the generation of cell-specific proteins. Because of the time necessary to generate these proteins, the earliest change that can be seen after an intravenous injection is in one hour, with the maximum effect seen in eight hours. Because of this delayed onset, steroids should not be considered the first line of defense in life-threatening allergic reactions.

Typically, parenteral steroids are administered subcutaneously, intramuscularly, or intralesionally. The intralesional route really is subcutaneous (sublesional) administration, as it is very difficult to give intralesional steroids with a needle and syringe. Intralesional steroids can cause as many side effects as subcutaneous or intramuscular steroids.

Aside from cases of life-threatening allergic reactions, parenteral steroids should have limited usage in the management of allergic skin disease. Regardless of the product used, the precise daily dose released and the duration of action are extremely variable. With repositol forms, HPAA suppression far outlasts the anti-inflammatory duration of the drug. Parenteral steroids should be reserved for those patients in whom anti-inflammatory therapy is required for two weeks or less, once or twice a year. If more frequent or constant therapy is required, oral steroids should be used. Some owners will report that oral medications do not work as well as injections. This is usually due to an insufficient oral dose of medication and can be corrected by increasing the dose or changing the drug. If parenteral drugs are truly the only effective steroid for the animal, the long-term prognosis is very guarded.

Antihistamines

Antihistamines in a strict sense are not true anti-inflammatory drugs, but they can be beneficial in the treatment of allergic disorders. Antihistamines are compounds with varied chemical structures that are able to antagonize some of the actions of histamines. These drugs work by competitively antagonizing histamines at the receptor site on cell membranes. Two classes of histamine receptors, namely H_1 and H_2, are recognized. H_1 receptors mediate the classic allergic changes seen with histamine, while the H_2 receptors mediate gastric acid secretion. H_2 receptors also are found in membranes of mast cells, basophils, and lymphocytes. Endogenous histamine stimulates the receptors in these cells in a negative feedback fashion such that further histamine release is inhibited.

All H_1 antihistamines have some local anesthetic property and some enhance the effects of sympathomimetic catecholamines, such as epinephrine. Sedation is a common side effect, but hyperexcitability can occur in sensitive animals or at high doses. A list of the various H_1 antihistamines is shown in Table 6–2. Cimetidine (Tagamet) is the commonly used H_2 antihistamine. By itself, this drug has no dermatologic applications, and it could increase the severity of allergic reactions by inhibiting the negative feedback mechanism of histamines on mast cells. It has been suggested that the combination of an H_1 blocker and cimetidine gives better results than those obtained with just the H_1 blocker. Cimetidine is given at a dose of 6.6 mg/kg every 8 hours. The frequency of administration coupled with the expense of this drug have limited its clinical use in allergic disease.

As can be seen from Table 6–2, a wide variety of H_1 antihistamines are available, each with a slightly different effect. Hydroxyzine is classified as a true ataractic drug that has the psychotropic effect of producing calmness without depression or clouded consciousness. Additionally, this drug has antihistaminic effects and can stabilize mast cell membranes. Hydroxyzine has had limited applicability in the past because of its expense, but it now is available in a generic form.

In a study on the effectiveness of nonsteroidal anti-inflammatory drugs on canine pruritus, Scott found that H_1 antihistamines were more effective than was earlier believed. In this study, a good response was one in which the drug satisfactorily controlled the pruritus, such that no other medications were necessary. A moderate

TABLE 6–2. H_1 Antagonists for Use in the Dog

DRUG CLASS	DRUG NAME	ORAL DOSAGE
Alkylamine	Chlorpheniramine	2–12 mg b.i.d. or t.i.d.
Ethanolamine	Diphenhydramine	2–4 mg/kg t.i.d.
	Dimenhydrinate	8 mg/kg t.i.d.
Ethylenediamine	Pyrilamine	1–2 mg/kg b.i.d.
	Tripelennamine	1–1.5 mg/kg b.i.d.
Piperazine	Hydroxyzine	2.2 mg/kg t.i.d.
	Meclizine	25 mg s.i.d.
Piperidine	Cyproheptadine	0.3–2.0 mg/kg b.i.d.
Phenothiazine	Promethazine	0.2–1.0 mg/kg b.i.d. or t.i.d.
	Trimeprazine	1–2 mg/kg t.i.d.

response indicated a significant reduction in itch but the residual pruritus required additional therapy. H_1 antihistamines produced good results in 10 of 45 dogs (22.2 percent) and a moderate response in another 19 dogs (43.2 percent). The percentage of good and moderate responses for the drugs studied were as follows: chlorpheniramine, 8.9/8.9; diphenhydramine, 6.7/15.6; and hydroxyzine, 6.7/17.8. A dog that does not respond to one class of drug could respond to another, so all classes of H_1 antihistamines should be tried before concluding that antihistamines are ineffective.

As was discussed before, antihistamines can be used in conjunction with steroids to decrease the dose of the steroids. Combining these drugs with other nonsteroidal drugs can further decrease the steroid dose.

Nonsteroidal Anti-inflammatory Drugs

A large number of nonsteroidal anti-inflammatory drugs (NSAIDs) exists and more are being developed. For most of these agents, little information about their clinical pharmacology in small animals is available. While the exact mode of action for each of these drugs varies, they all inhibit prostaglandin synthesis. The salicylates also depress prostaglandin actions and inhibit the formation of kinins. Vitamin E and Derm Caps (DVM) also inhibit leukotriene synthesis.

Most NSAIDs are highly protein-bound, which gives prolonged effects but also can cause pharmacokinetic interactions by displacing other agents from their protein binding sites. Gastrointestinal ulceration and bleeding can occur as a result of the irritation of these drugs, because these drugs decrease the protective prostaglandin production, or both. Bleeding disorders, nephrotoxicity, and drug eruptions also can be seen with many of the agents.

Aspirin and phenylbutazone are the two NSAIDs that receive widest use in the dog, and neither is particularly effective in treating allergic skin disease. Aspirin at a dose of 25 mg/kg every 8 hours produced good results in only one dog in Scott's study. At this dose, bleeding tendencies can occur.

Recently, a fatty acid nutritional supplement (Derm Caps) was marketed, and this product appears to have significant NSAID activity. The eicosapentaenoic acid (EPA) appears to be the most significant of all ingredients. This fatty acid can shift prostaglandin and leukotriene synthesis away from the two-series of prostaglandins and the four-series of leukotrienes. The other prostaglandins and leukotrienes that are formed appear to have less of an inflammatory potential.

In a study by one author (WHM), 18.3 percent of the allergic dogs showed a good response to Derm Caps, while another 17.2 percent showed a moderate response. Scott noted a good response in 11.1 percent of his dogs and a moderate response in another 11.1 percent. Other investigators have not had equally good results.

In an initial study on the effects of fatty acid supplements in allergic dogs, Lloyd found that 62.5 percent of his patients improved with evening primrose oil (EPO) supplementation. The seborrheic signs of the dogs improved markedly, although their pruritus was unaffected. The addition of EPA to the evening primrose oil had no positive effects. In more recent work with EPO/EPA supplementation that contains vitamins and minerals (EfaVet), Lloyd reported results to be excellent in 18 percent, good in 76 percent, and none in 6 percent after six weeks. This improvement included both seborrheic signs and pruritus.

The studies cited above show that fatty acid supplements containing EPO/EPA can be beneficial in the treatment of allergic disorders. As this mode of therapy is relatively new, further studies are necessary to clarify the effectiveness of these and other fatty acid supplements. These supplements may also allow the clinician to use lower doses of glucocorticoids.

MISCELLANEOUS AGENTS

Gold Salt Therapy (Chrysotherapy)

Chrysotherapy is used in the treatment of rheumatoid arthritis and certain autoimmune skin diseases. Among their effects, gold compounds can stabilize lysosomal membranes, decrease migration and phagocytic activity of macrophages and neutrophils, inhibit prostaglandin synthesis, and suppress immunoglobulin synthesis. These effects would be valuable in the treatment of allergic disorders.

Aurothioglucose (Solganal) is the most widely used gold compound in veterinary medicine, and it is administered at a dose of 1 mg/kg IM once weekly after two test doses. A lag phase of 6 to 12 weeks is common. In veterinary medicine, reported side effects are few, but nephrotoxicity and bone marrow suppression can be seen. During the induction phase of therapy, a urinalysis should be run weekly and a hemogram should be done bimonthly.

Although the drug itself is relatively inexpensive, chrysotherapy can be expensive because of the weekly veterinary visits and the cost of the laboratory tests. The authors are unaware of any reports about the use of chrysotherapy in allergic animals, but this mode of therapy has some potential.

Cytotoxic Immunosuppressants

In veterinary dermatology, the alkylating agent cyclophosphamide (Cytoxan) and the antimetabolite azathioprine (Imuran) are the two most commonly used cytotoxic immunosuppressants. These agents, among their other effects, decrease antibody production and the number of leukocytes. Although both of these drugs can cause a significant leukopenia, this is more likely with cyclophosphamide. In addition, a sterile hemorrhagic cystitis can be caused by cyclophosphamide. Azathioprine is a less potent drug with a very low incidence of side effects. Because of its relative safety, azathioprine is the dermatologic drug of choice.

Azathioprine is administered at a dose of 2.2 mg/kg orally once daily or every other day. Hemograms are monitored every two weeks. Immunosuppressant therapy rarely is used for allergic disorders. The authors are aware of patients that are being managed with azathioprine because no other form of therapy was effective. Obviously, this therapy was a last resort.

Orgotein

Orgotein (Palosein) is a copper-zinc superoxide dismutase approved for use in the dog. Superoxide dismutases work by inactivating destructive superoxide radicals released during inflammation. They may also prevent disruption of lysosomal membranes. Side effects appear to be few, but because orgotein is weakly immunogenic, anaphylaxis has been reported following its repeated administration.

Although approved for the treatment of generalized conditions in the dog, Orgotein is very expensive and the authors have not had any first-hand experience with it. This product's expense limits its applicability.

Vitamin E

Vitamin E is a nonsteroidal anti-inflammatory drug that also blocks lipid peroxidation of polyunsaturated fatty acids. This decreases the amount of free radicals and hydroperoxides formed during the inflammatory process. Vitamin E at doses of 200 to 400 IU b.i.d. has proven to be effective in the treatment of canine discoid lupus erythematosus and epidermolysis bullosa, but it appears to be of little benefit in the treatment of allergic disorders.

Psychotropic Drugs

This group of drugs exerts an effect upon the mind, and some of the drugs have more direct cutaneous effects. Although initiated by disease, pruritus can be self-perpetuating and habit-forming. This is especially true in the small nervous breeds. Mind-altering drugs can help break this habit.

Phenothiazines

In human medicine, chlorpromazine is used as a psychotropic drug that not only has central effects but also has antihistaminic, anticholinergic, and alpha-adrenergic blocking effects. Sedation can be marked. In small animals, acetylpromazine (acepromazine) is used more widely than chlorpromazine, and it also has antihistaminic and sedative effects. Acepromazine is administered at a dose of 0.55 to 2.2 mg/kg PO, while chlorpromazine can be given at 3.3 mg/kg PO. Because of the size of the tablets and variations in absorption, the effects of acepromazine seem to be "all or nothing"—either no effect is noted or marked sedation occurs. The marked sedation may be tolerated for a few days while diagnostic tests are scheduled but is unacceptable for long-term management. Phenothiazines should not be used in animals with seizure disorders, and long-term administration can result in photosensitization or a drug eruption.

Tricyclic Antidepressants

Tricyclic antidepressants are structurally related to the phenothiazine group and are some of the most potent antihistamines known. These drugs inhibit the activity of histamine by blocking both the H_1 and H_2 receptors, and they have anticholinergic activity. Amitriptyline (Elavil) is the drug used in veterinary medicine for behavior modification. Amitriptyline is administered orally to dogs at a dose of 1 to 2 mg/kg once daily. The authors are unaware of any reports regarding the use of amitriptyline in the management of allergic disease but, because of the physiologic effects of this drug, it has some potential especially in the nervous dog. In humans, there are many contraindications for the use of amitriptyline, so it is advisable to consult a pharmacology text before using the drug.

Miscellaneous Psychotropic Drugs

Sedatives, tranquilizers, and barbiturates all have been used to relieve pruritus. However, depression can be severe, so these agents have little use for long-term management.

Miscellaneous Agents

Cromolyn sodium has no anti-inflammatory effects but rather inhibits the degranulation of sensitized mast cells. The drug is administered by inhalation because gastrointestinal absorption is poor. In small animals, the drug is toxic and cannot be used.

The authors have used experimental mast cell stabilizers given orally. These drugs were very effective in the management of pruritus but are not currently available. Presently, there is renewed interest in this type of drug for dogs.

7 Food Hypersensitivity

INTRODUCTION

Adverse reactions to foods can be abnormal clinical responses to the ingestion of a food or food additive. Adverse reactions may have an immunologic or a nonimmunologic basis. In humans, nonallergic reactions are much more common than allergic reactions; most likely this is true in veterinary medicine as well. The terminology used to describe adverse reactions to foods is confusing because of the variety of interpretations. A standard nonmenclature to describe adverse reactions to foods has been proposed as follows:

Food Hypersensitivity: An immunologic reaction resulting from the ingestion of a food or food additive.

Food Intolerance: An abnormal physiologic response to an ingestant of an idiosyncratic, metabolic, pharmacologic, or toxic nature.

Food Idiosyncrasy: An abnormal response to an ingestant, resembling hypersensitivity but not involving immune mechanisms.

A common manifestation of food intolerance is diarrhea associated with the ingestion of cow's milk by a lactase-deficient individual. An example of a food idiosyncrasy is the development of urticaria after the ingestion of wine, egg whites, strawberries, shellfish, tomatoes, citrus fruit, or alcohol. These ingestants can cause nonimmunologic histamine release in some individuals. On a clinical basis, it is impossible to distinguish between a food hypersensitivity, intolerance, and idiosyncrasy. Dietary elimination and challenge testing may incriminate a certain food but do not define the mechanism. To make the firm diagnosis of a food hypersensitivity, evidence of immunologic reactivity must be found.

Adverse reactions to food can be manifested by cutaneous, respiratory, gastrointestinal, neurologic, and hematologic signs. Signs may be restricted to one organ system or may involve multiple organ systems. Within one organ system, the signs of an adverse food reaction are not specific. When they affect the skin, food hypersensitivities can mimic any other form of hypersensitivity disease, and thus the diagnosis can be excluded only by investigation.

PATHOGENESIS

The gastrointestinal tract is protected from injury by a number of immunologic and nonimmunologic mechanisms. Immunologic protection is provided by local, humoral, and cell-mediated immunity and mast cell activation. The humoral and cell-mediated responses appear to be initiated in the Peyer's patches. Sensitized cells circulate and return to the lamina propria of the bowel wall. Local antibody production typically involves IgA and IgM, with IgA predominating. Cells producing IgG and IgE can also be identified, but their numbers in adults are very small. These immunoglobulins are used as protection against microorganisms and parasites and also control the absorption of antigens.

In food hypersensitivities, antibodies against specific food antigens can be found in the serum and bowel secretions. Levels of all classes of immunoglobulins can be found. The significance of the circulating levels of IgA and IgG directed against foods is uncertain, since they can be found not only in patients with food hypersensitivities but also in normal individuals and in those with other disorders.

Type I hypersensitivity reactions have been documented in food hypersensitivity. The IgE produced in response to a food antigen can sensitize bowel mast cells or mast cells anywhere in the body. There is also evidence of type III and type IV hypersensitivity reactions to foods, but the findings are inconsistent. Until proven otherwise, it would be best to consider that the signs of a food hypersensitivity can be due to a type I, III, or IV hypersensitivity reaction.

PREVALENCE

The true incidence of adverse reactions to foods in animals is unknown. In dermatology, food hypersensitivity is the third most common allergic disease of the dog and the second most common in the cat. In the dog, the reported incidence varies from 1 percent of all dermatology cases to 23 percent of cases of nonseasonal allergic dermatitis. In a study by Baker of 82 dogs with nonseasonal allergic dermatitis, 18 percent showed a 10 to 50 percent improvement in their signs with food deprivation, while 21 percent improved from 51 to 90 percent. Obviously, food hypersensitivity can occur in conjunction with other allergic conditions. White reported that 23 percent of his patients with a food hypersensitivity also had some other allergic condition. Food hypersensitivity can be difficult to document in an animal with multiple forms of allergy.

No estimate of the incidence of the nondermatologic signs associated with food hypersensitivity can be made, although it has been estimated that between 10 and 15 percent of animals with dermatologic signs have concurrent gastrointestinal signs. Some claim that the incidence of concurrent gastrointestinal signs is much higher if the owner is carefully questioned about the occurrence of flatus, borborygmus, and subtle bowel changes. The authors believe that the incidence of concurrent bowel disease is much lower than that reported, having also recognized seizure disorders, cystitis, and respiratory disease in dogs with food hypersensitivity. The systemic signs disappeared with food deprivation and recurred with dietary challenge. In these cases, an immunologic abnormality was not documented, so the systemic signs could have been due to a food idiosyncrasy.

ETIOLOGIC AGENTS

Virtually any food or food additive can cause an adverse reaction. In humans, food idiosyncrasy mimicking food hypersensitivity has been noted with a number of different ingestants. Scombroid fish (such as tuna and mackerel) can contain large amounts of histamine if it is spoiled or stored at high temperatures. A variety of foods contain such vasoactive amines as tyramine, tryptamine (cheese), phenylethylamine (chocolate), dopamine, norepinephrine, serotonin, and histamine. Wine, egg whites, strawberries, shellfish, tomatoes, citrus fruits, and alcohol can cause nonimmunologic mast cell degranulation in certain individuals. With the exception of scombroid fish, such foods are usually not fed to animals, so the incidence of food idiosyncrasies should be low.

In humans, common agents of food hypersensitivity are peanuts, nuts, seafood, eggs, seeds, milk, chocolate, barley, rice, wheat, citrus fruits, melons, bananas, tomatoes, spinach, corn, potatoes, and soybeans. In some food groups, especially the legumes and seafoods, allergy to one member of the group may result in allergy to another member because of antigen cross-reactivity. Within a species, animal products tend not to cross-react. For example, a person allergic to cow's milk often can eat beef and inhale cow dander. Cooking and digestion can destroy the antigenicity of some foods and expose new antigens in others.

Individuals allergic to beef obviously should avoid veal, but other bovine products such as liver, sweetbreads, and gelatin should also be suspect. Cow's milk is a complex food that contains over 30 separate proteins. The β-lactoglobulin fraction is the most allergenic, followed by casein, lactalbumin, and bovine serum albumin. Whole milk, skim milk, and powdered milk are all equally antigenic. Although milk and milk products (such as cheese) are easily recognized on food labels, milk components such as casein, caseinate, lactose, and whey are common ingredients that may go unrecognized.

Cow's milk, beef, lamb, pork, chicken, rabbit, horsemeat, fish, and eggs have been reported to cause food hypersensitivity in dogs and cats. In the dog, wheat, corn, rice, flour, potatoes, soybeans, and kidney beans have also been associated with food hypersensitivity. In most instances, the exact food causing the problem remains unidentified because the owner is unable or unwilling to go through the laborious task of provocative challenge testing.

When examining the diet of an animal, one has to be careful of hidden allergens. Mixed vegetable oils can contain any number of oils. Animal fats, meat by-products, and meat and bone meal could be from cow, pig, or chicken. Natural vitamin A products may contain fish. Food starch or modified food starch could be from wheat, corn, sorghum, arrowroot, tapioca, or potato. Some medications may contain a binder such as calcium or magnesium stearate made from the stearic acid of pork, beef, or lamb fat. In addition, flavoring agents are usually not specified.

CLINICAL PRESENTATION

Animals with food hypersensitivities typically are presented with perennial problems. Since a food hypersensitivity can start at any time of the year, the signs may start during a peak pollen period and mimic atopic disease. The authors have seen dogs with seasonal or episodic food hypersensitivities. Seasonal food hypersensitivity could be associated with the ingestion of seasonal allergens (crabs, fresh fruit, vegetables) or could be due to allergy exacerbation by pollens. Dogs can have multiple forms of allergy simultaneously. For example, a dog's perennial borderline food allergy may become symptomatic when its atopic disease flares. This flare can be explained by cross-reactive antigens in the pollen and food or by the threshold phenomenon. In humans, cross-reactions between inhaled and ingested molds, between ragweed and melons or bananas, between birch pollen and carrots, parsnips, apples, potatoes or hazelnuts; and between grass pollens and cereals have been recognized. Exposure to the pollen would aggravate the food hypersensitivity. Some animals can have an atopic condition and a food hypersensitivity simultaneously—with neither significant enough by itself to cause pruritus. If both occur simultaneously, the dog may itch. Elimination of either the food or the pollen factor causes the other allergic condition to become asymptomatic. The authors have not seen any cross-reactions between foods and pollens but have recognized patients with subclinical food hypersensitivity aggravated by pollen allergies.

Episodic food hypersensitivity occurs when the animal eats the offending agent periodically. In these cases, the index of suspicion for a food hypersensitivity can be very low. The animal that shows repetitive but episodic signs of allergic dermatitis should be suspected of having food hypersensitivity. The owner should be questioned very carefully about table foods, treats, and so forth given to the animal. Clinical signs usually become manifest within several hours of ingestion, but if the antigen is a digested protein or one created by bacterial conversion, signs can occur up to 24 hours later. With a late onset of signs, the effects of causative food may be obscured by those of foods ingested in the interim. A daily log book is very helpful. The authors have seen cases of periodic food hypersensitivity when pizza was fed to a dog or when a cat ate a mouse.

The age of onset is variable. Food hypersensitivity can occur at any age even in the young animal less than one year old. Walton reported that 68 percent of his patients with food hypersensitivities had been exposed to the allergen for over two years before the clinical signs developed. If signs occur with the first exposure, a food idiosyncrasy is most probable.

The cutaneous signs of a food hypersensitivity are not specific and can mimic many other dermatologic conditions. In the dog, the more common clinical presentations are generalized pruritus with or without lesions, atopy or flea allergy-patterned pruritus (Fig. 7–1), and urticaria. Less common findings are recurrent episodes of acute moist dermatitis, recurrent pyodermas, otitis externa, seborrhea (Fig. 7–2), and generalized hyperemia. In the cat, the more common signs of food allergy are facial pruritus (Fig. 7–3) or miliary dermatitis. Less frequent presentations are generalized pruritus, atopic-like pruritus, and psychogenic alopecia (Fig. 7–4). Secondary pyodermas can be superimposed on the primary skin signs. Gastrointestinal or other systemic manifestations may accompany the skin signs.

Following sensitization, symptoms should occur following every subsequent exposure even if the allergen is present in small amounts. The degree of sensitivity varies, so some animals may not show signs unless large quantities are ingested. If the animal is sensitive to several allergens, ingestion of small quantities of each allergen may trigger clinical signs. Multiple sensitivities to ingested allergens appear to be rare in the dog and cat.

Although the onset of clinical signs is rapid, improvement is not immediate following withholding of the food. Chronically pruritic animals have altered cutaneous sensibilities such that many cutaneous feelings (e.g., pressure) are interpreted as itch. Secondary skin changes, such as seborrhea or pyoderma, increase the itchiness

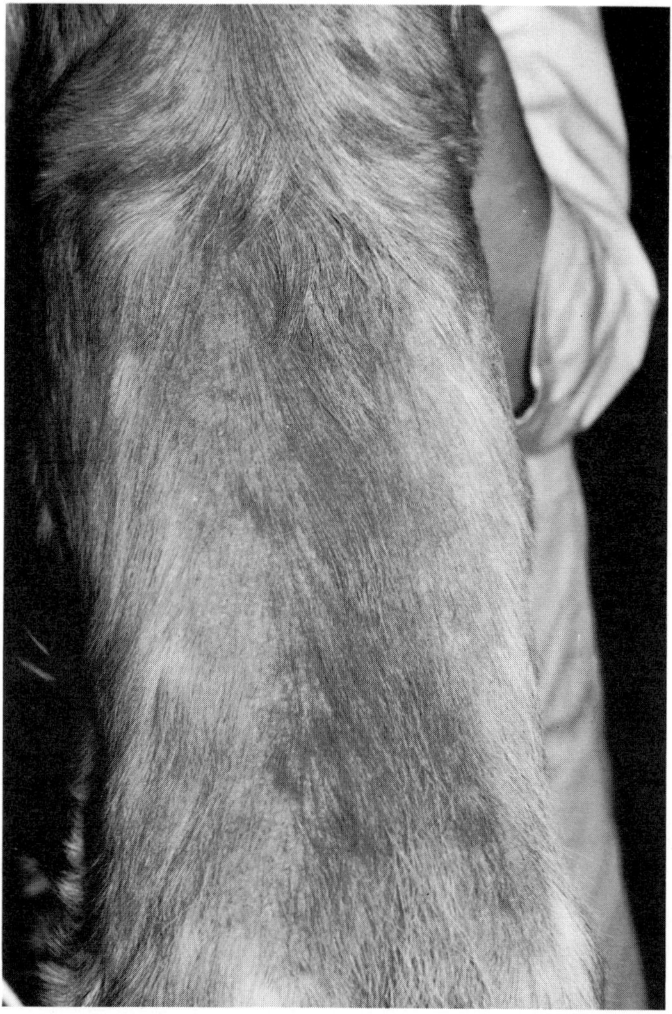

FIGURE 7–1. Traumatic hair loss over the lower back.

of the skin so that the animal may continue to itch even if the offending food is avoided. In the animal that does not have chronically diseased skin, withdrawal of the food usually causes the pruritus to cease in approximately 48 to 72 hours.

With food hypersensitivity, the animal's response to glucocorticoids is variable. Animals with food hypersensitivities do not usually respond as well to glucocorticoid therapy as those with other types

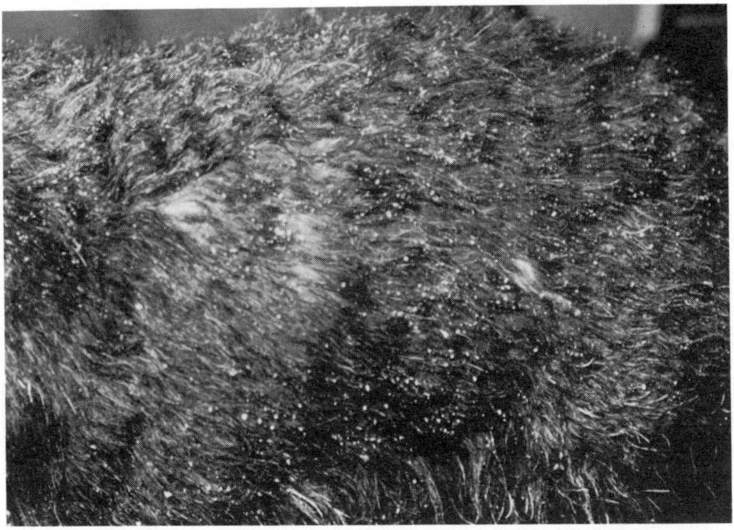

FIGURE 7–2. Seborrhea sicca due to a food hypersensitivity.

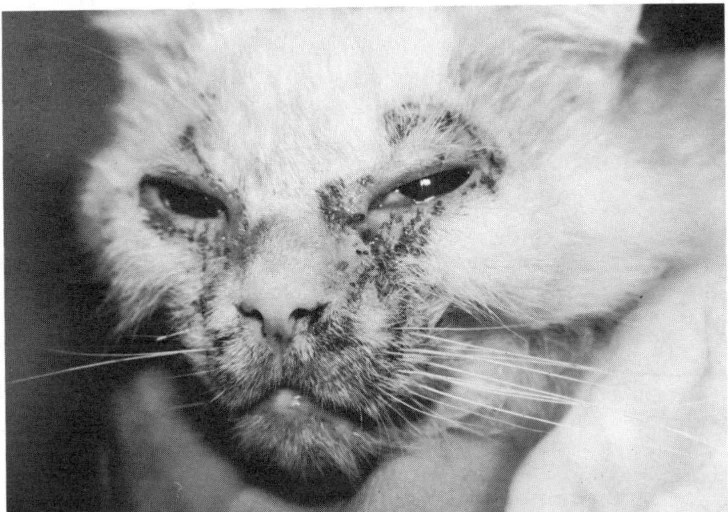

FIGURE 7–3. Facial pruritus induced by a food hypersensitivity.

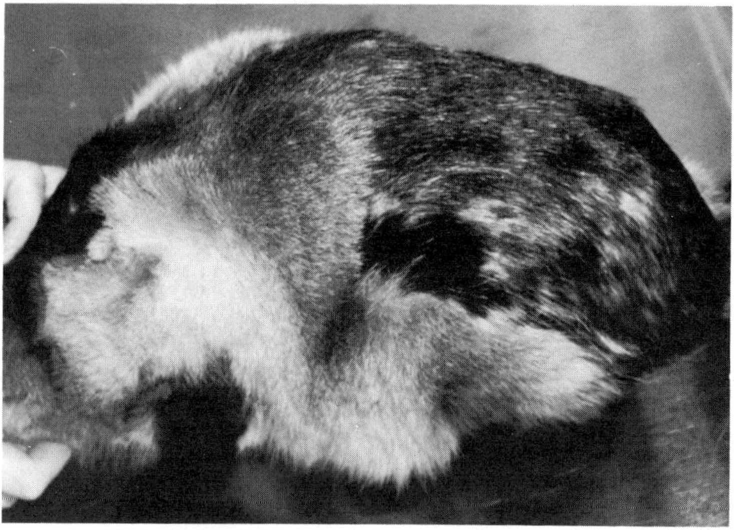

FIGURE 7–4. **Traumatic hair loss over the lower back of a cat.**

of allergies. This steroid resistance could be due to the severity or chronicity of the hypersensitivity or could indicate a complicated immunologic basis. Response to glucocorticoid therapy can be a useful diagnostic test. An allergic cat with facial pruritus that does not respond to adequate steroid therapy is a strong candidate for the diagnosis of a food hypersensitivity. If the animal does respond to glucocorticoid therapy, the diagnosis of food hypersensitivity cannot be dismissed.

DIAGNOSTIC APPROACH

Food hypersensitivity can mimic any other allergic condition and, depending on the history, should always be considered. To distinguish between a food hypersensitivity and a food idiosyncrasy, evidence of immunologic reactivity must be found. In veterinary medicine, the demonstration of an immunologic response to a food is difficult, if not impossible. Presently, food hypersensitivity is demonstrated by dietary manipulation, although elimination diets and food rechallenge do not determine the allergic basis. Repeated flares with exposure to small amounts of food strongly support the allergic basis.

Elimination Diets

Before dietary elimination is started, the owner must understand that everything the animal eats is suspect and must be avoided. One indiscretion by any family member or by the pet can void the test up to that point. Animals that hunt or scavenge cannot be tested unless they are confined.

If the animal has concurrent atopic disease, or flea allergy dermatitis, or both, the avoidance diet should not be started until the flea or pollen season is over if possible. If the avoidance diet is started during the peak pollen or flea season, any food-associated decrease in the animal's level of pruritus may be impossible to detect. If the animal has a secondary pyoderma, that should be resolved first. Resolution of the pyoderma will usually relieve the animal's pruritus, and if antibiotics and the diet are begun simultaneously, it will be impossible to judge the diet's effect.

Avoidance can be accomplished by starvation or by feeding a restrictive or hypoallergenic diet. Since prolonged fasting is unacceptable to most owners, restrictive diets are used. A short period of fasting coupled with the use of cathartics may hasten the animal's response. Because commercial pet foods contain similar ingredients, switching from one brand or type of commercial food to another is not adequate. Special foods must be prepared. Water can contain fungi, algae, and other allergenic substances; therefore, distilled water should be used for cooking and drinking when the household's water supply is from a well.

The restrictive diet must be tailored to the animal's typical diet and the frequency and nature of snack foods. Foods given with some regularity are suspect and should be avoided. If the animal has eaten a food, such as lamb, very infrequently, it can be used for the test diet. For the dog, a protein and a carbohydrate source must be selected, while only a protein source is needed for the cat. Brown rice and potatoes are good carbohydrate sources. Lamb, fish, rabbit, and venison are good protein sources; but chicken or turkey can be used for some dogs. In the cat, lamb is the best choice, but veal, chicken, and turkey may also be acceptable, depending on the cat's previous eating habits. Because sudden dietary changes can cause gastrointestinal signs in animals, the special diet should be introduced slowly over three to four days.

Most cats will accept baby food, and thus the diet is simplified for the cat owner. If the cat craves something to chew on, overcooked meat can be added to the baby food. Overcooked lamb can be as chewy as any commercial cat food.

For dogs, home cooking will be necessary unless the dog is very small and the feeding of baby food is practical. Hypoallergenic foods are available commercially (d/d, Hill's), but the authors prefer not to use commercial foods during the test period. White reported that 54 percent of his patients that responded to home-cooked lamb and rice would experience a flare in their condition when given d/d. The reason for this is unknown.

The rice or potatoes are boiled and mixed with the protein source at a ratio of 4:1 or 2:1. Extra water should be added to the ration at each feeding because these diets tend to cause constipation. The protein source can be boiled, broiled, or baked. If fish is used, water-packed tuna fish can be fed without additional preparation. For large dogs, white types of fish can be used. Fillets can be prepared in standard fashion or whole fish can be cooked in a pressure cooker to dissolve the bones.

The hypoallergenic diet is fed at the same volume as the normal ration, and the animal is given free access to fresh water. In some animals, the amount of food will have to be increased to satisfy their hunger. While the diet is being fed, the animal should not receive anything else. No table foods, rawhide chew sticks, dog bones, and unnecessary medications should be given. Dogs that need to chew can have unflavored nylon bones. If a medication is necessary, such as heartworm preventative, an unflavored form should be used.

Most food-hypersensitive animals will show some response to the diet in two weeks. If the skin was severely diseased at the beginning of the diet, the response may be slow, and the diet may have to be fed for three to four weeks. If the symptoms do not subside at all with the diet, the diagnosis of a food hypersensitivity is not acceptable. If the animal becomes normal with the diet, a food allergy is strongly suspect. If the symptoms decrease significantly but not completely, the animal may have a food hypersensitivity concurrent with some other disease, or the improvement may be coincidental. When improvement is noted, the animal should be challenged with its old diet including treats to see if the signs recur. If the signs do not recur with challenge, the improvement was coincidental. If the signs recur, a food hypersensitivity or idiosyncrasy has been documented, and the hypoallergenic diet should be reinstituted. One singular challenge test supports but does not confirm the diagnosis of a food hypersensitivity, since immunologic reactivity has not been documented.

Other Diagnostic Techniques

Various in vivo and in vitro tests are available in human medicine to aid in the diagnosis of a food hypersensitivity. Cytotoxic tests have not been shown to be reliable or reproducible and should not be used. Basophil or leukocyte histamine release assays are specific and reproducible tests, although they are untried in veterinary medicine, and their technical difficulties limit their usefulness. Direct skin testing and serologic testing are used most frequently.

Skin testing and serologic testing are used to identify specific IgE antibodies to a food. In humans, the correlation between positive skin test results and clinical sensitivity is excellent if pure allergen extracts are used. Until standardization is available for all food antigens, the reliability of skin test results depends on the quality of the test antigens used. The results of serologic tests are similarly affected by the purity of the test antigen. Both of these tests indicate the presence of an antibody that may or may not be clinically significant. Clinical significance must be proved by provocative challenge. In veterinary medicine, skin testing remains unproven. McDougal reported that he found RAST to be unreliable for testing food hypersensitivity in dogs.

Skin biopsies are of little diagnostic value. One usually sees a superficial perivascular dermatitis with some hyperplastic epidermal changes; these changes are common to most hypersensitivity disorders. Presently, hypoallergenic diet testing is the most specific test for food hypersensitivity in animals.

TREATMENT

The therapy for food hypersensitivity is simple—avoid the food. This is more complex than it sounds, however, because the offending food must be identified. Provocative challenge testing is necessary to identify the allergen and this testing can be time-consuming. The provocative challenge testing is done by adding one pure food to the restrictive diet every fifth day. Table food works nicely for most of the testing. Flour or crackers can be used to test the various grains. Only one food is added at a time. If the signs recur or intensify during the challenge period, the animal may not be able to tolerate that particular food and it should be discontinued. Once the skin has returned to the prechallenge state, the next food is added until the entire list of test foods (Table 7–1) is completed. Although most dogs and cats have singular sensitivities, multiple ones can occur.

Many animals with food hypersensitivities can eat some specially selected commercial foods. The list of ingredients of the various foods is compared with the results of the provocative challenge testing, and a hypoallergenic commercial food is selected. If the animal cannot tolerate it, the food either has some hidden allergen or the animal is also allergic to additives, artificial flavors, dyes, or preservatives. In the authors' experience this additional allergy is

TABLE 7–1. Foods for Challenge Testing

Beef	Corn
Liver	Soy
Pork	Wheat
Chicken	Brewer's yeast
Veal	Milk
Lamb	Egg
Fish	

TABLE 7–2. Maintenance Hypoallergenic Diet for Dogs and Cats

4 oz	Lamb
1 cup	Cooked rice
1 tsp	Vegetable oil
1½ tsp	Dicalcium phosphate
Balanced, unflavored vitamin/mineral supplement	
Yield: 2/3 pound (530 kcal)	

(From Lewis, L.D., Morris, M.L., Jr., and Hand, M.S.: Small Animal Clinical Nutrition (3rd ed): Topeka, KS, Mark Morris Associates, 1987.)

rare, so a hidden allergen is most likely. Another similar commercial food should be tried.

Some owners are unwilling or unable to complete the provocative exposure testing. All animals should be tested for cow's milk, and the dog at least should be tested for beef. Fish should be tried in the cat. If the animal reacts to one or both of these test antigens, a commercial food that does not contain that agent can be tried and can usually be tolerated. If the animal does not react to either of these tests, commercial foods should not be given.

When animals cannot eat over-the-counter commercial foods, veterinary prescription diets such as d/d can be tried or home cooking can be continued. D/d is adequate for both dogs and cats. With home cooking, the diet must be supplemented with fats, vitamins, and minerals to assure nutritional adequacy (Table 7–2). To assure good taurine levels for cats, one-half teaspoon of clam juice should be added to the food daily.

Animals with food hypersensitivities can develop future sensitivities, even to lamb, which is erroneously thought to be nonallergenic. If this happens, the whole provocative challenge test can be repeated, or a new diet based on the previous list can be tried. A more troublesome problem occurs when a safe food cannot be found or when the animal refuses to eat the hypoallergenic food. Medical management is then necessary. This can be very difficult especially if the animal responds poorly to glucocorticoids. One author (WHM) has had to euthanize two cats that refused to eat anything except what they were allergic to.

In humans, especially in children, spontaneous remission of food hypersensitivity has been recognized. This phenomenon may be the result of the development of immunologic tolerance as the immune system or the digestive system matures. These findings have not been reported in animals. Challenge with the offending food every six months or so will indicate whether or not spontaneous remission occurs in animals.

8 Allergic Contact Dermatitis

INTRODUCTION

Substances that contact the skin can cause a dermatitis by both allergic and nonallergic mechanisms. Allergic contact dermatitis and nonallergic (irritant contact) dermatitis are clinically similar, and both types can exist simultaneously. Contact dermatitis of either type is uncommon in the dog and rare in the cat.

In acute contact dermatitis, the affected skin is red, warm, and usually pruritic. Papules and plaques may be seen if there has not been too much damage from self-trauma. Depending on the severity of the reaction, vesicles or bullae may form. Because of the nature of animal skin, these lesions are very transient and often are not seen. In chronic cases, the skin is thickened, lichenified, crusted, and usually hyperpigmented. Secondary pyodermas and seborrheic changes are common.

IRRITANT CONTACT DERMATITIS

Irritant contact dermatitis is caused by a direct chemical assault of an agent on the skin. Although no good studies exist in veterinary medicine to document the incidence of irritant contact dermatitis, it is thought that this form of contact dermatitis is much more common than the allergic form.

Many substances will damage the skin when applied at a high enough concentration for a sufficient period of time. Primary irritants may be divided according to their known actions: acids (HCl), bases (NaOH), organic solvents (benzene), detergents (sodium lauryl sulfate), desiccants (calcium dioxide), and oxidizers (chlorine). Almost any substance can cause irritation in an individual depending on the conditions of application and the individual's degree of sensitivity.

With strong irritants, the reaction will occur immediately after the first exposure; all animals exposed to the irritant should develop signs of disease. With milder irritants such as detergents, repeated contact may be necessary before signs become evident. With these milder irritants, most but not all of the animals exposed to the substance will show signs of disease.

In allergic contact dermatitis, application of dilute solutions of the allergen will cause reactions. This is not true in irritant contact dermatitis, which is highly concentration-dependent. While there is considerable variation among individuals and areas of the body susceptible to irritation, if the agent is applied under the appropriate conditions, all individuals will react.

For irritation reactions to occur, relatively large amounts of the agent must penetrate the skin. Pre-existing disease can diminish the barrier function of the epidermis and allow greater penetration of the irritant. Accordingly, irritant contact dermatitis may be superimposed on another allergic disorder. Some substances, such as cement, can be both irritants and allergens.

ALLERGIC CONTACT DERMATITIS

Allergic contact dermatitis is caused by a type IV hypersensitivity reaction to an allergen. Because of the immunologic basis of this disorder, only a limited number of individuals in an exposed population will develop signs of disease. Unless the allergen is also an irritant, the reaction will not occur at initial exposure, regardless of the concentration. Repeated or continuous challenge is necessary for sensitization to occur and for the signs to develop. The best known example of allergic contact dermatitis is the poison ivy/poison oak reaction in humans. The sensitivity is acquired and requires repeated exposure. Nonsensitized individuals show no reaction to these plants. Sensitized individuals may be affected by cross-reactive antigens found in mangos and certain tree lacquers.

The contactant may be a complete allergen, a low molecular weight substance (hapten), or a photoallergen. Most contactants are simple chemicals, which are haptens. These agents must be conjugated to skin proteins before they become allergenic. Photoallergens also tend to be simple chemicals. In this case, the agent must be activated by the absorption of light before it can become a hapten. The reaction can occur only at sites exposed to light.

Pathogenesis

Allergic contact dermatitis is a type IV or delayed-type hypersensitivity reaction. The development of clinical sensitivity occurs in three phases. Initially, there is a refractory phase in which there is no evidence of skin disease or immunologic activity. This phase varies in length. Next, there is an incubation period in which an immunologic reaction (sensitization) occurs, yet the skin remains normal. This phase typically lasts five days. After the incubation period, the phase of hypersensitivity is reached. Application of the agent will then cause skin changes. Sensitivity is probably life-long, but reactivity will decrease if exposure is limited.

Epidermal Langerhans' cells play a pivotal role in the development of allergic contact dermatitis. Each Langerhans' cell possesses a central body with a lobulated nucleus and several dendritic branches that pass between keratinocytes in a radial fashion. Langerhans' cells cover most skin surfaces as a regularly distributed network, residing entirely within the epidermis. Langerhans' cells have a macrophage lineage, and they contribute via antigen presentation to the proliferation and clonal expansion of sensitized lymphocytes.

The antigen is carried to the regional lymph nodes draining the area of application, and sensitization occurs in these nodes. Sensitized T lymphocytes circulate throughout the body causing a generalized sensitivity usually in five days. After sensitization, the development of clinical lesions can occur anywhere the substance is applied, not just at the initial site of application. With re-exposure, lesions do not occur immediately but rather on the average in 24 to 48 hours. This latent period can vary from a few hours up to five days.

Prevalence

Contact dermatitis is uncommon in companion animals and, because of problems in the accurate differentiation between allergic contact and irritant contact dermatitis, the true incidence of allergic contact dermatitis is unknown. The incidence has been estimated to vary from 1 to 10 percent of dermatology cases, but the authors believe that allergic contact dermatitis occurs even less frequently. Most animals are exposed to a large number of potential contact allergens throughout their lives and never develop clinical sensitivity. This low incidence of sensitivity is explained by the protective nature of the pelage, or coat, and the poor capability of dogs and cats of developing type IV hypersensitivity reactions. However, dogs and cats can be sensitized, so there must be another explanation for the low incidence.

In humans, there is marked variation in the susceptibility to developing allergic contact dermatitis. Some patients are easily sensitized, while a small segment of the population cannot be sensitized even to potent agents such as dinitrochlorobenzene (DNCB). Experimental studies in humans indicate a trend toward genetic clustering. Patients capable of becoming sensitized are more likely to have children susceptible to sensitization than patients who are not easily sensitized. Patients sensitized to one chemical are more likely to become sensitized to another. There is evidence that certain strains of laboratory animals do possess a genetic predisposition to developing contact sensitivity. To date, there are no data to suggest that genetic factors are operative in companion animals.

In humans, contact allergic dermatitis is more common in patients with other chronic skin disorders. Abrasions and repeated minor trauma to the skin appear to aid in the initiation of contact hypersensitivity. Epidermal changes result in decreased barrier function, allowing increased permeability. Patients with atopic dermatitis have a relatively high incidence of contact hypersensitivity to drugs, although as a group, these people are more difficult to sensitize than normal control subjects. The relatively high incidence of drug sensitivity is the result of frequent applications of a wide variety of topical agents to inflamed skin.

Despite the possible genetic influence, what determines the onset of sensitivity remains a mystery. In humans, males have a higher incidence than females. The young and the elderly are more difficult to sensitize than young or middle-aged adults. Certain exogenous factors predispose to sensitization; for example, a seasonal variation is recognized. Skin that becomes dry during winter is more easily sensitized. Sweating during the summer can bring allergens from clothing in close contact with the skin. Repeated contact with the agent over large areas of the body favors sensitization. Application of the agent to damaged skin, at high concentrations, and under occlusion increases the penetration of the agent, which favors sensitization.

ETIOLOGIC AGENTS

The causes of contact allergy are many and varied; virtually any drug, chemical, or plant can cause sensitization. In humans, poison ivy/poison oak is a common contactant; but this is rare in the dog. In the dog, contact allergy has been reported to the oleoresin of certain plant pollens, jasmine blossoms (Lonicera), and the wandering Jew (*Tradescantia fluminensis*).

Topical medications often cause contact allergy in humans. Reactions are seen in animals, but the incidence is low probably because topical drugs are used infrequently. In humans, neomycin, benzocaine, ethylenediamine, and lanolin are very common sensitizers. In animals, neomycin is the most common agent. Topical products containing coal tars or insecticides are reported to cause sensitization; however, because these agents are irritants, the reaction may not be a true allergic phenomenon. With medications, the sensitization can be due to the drug, the vehicle (lanolin), or the preservatives (parabens, parachlorometaxylenol, dichlorophene, and so forth).

Other reported contact allergens in the dog include plastics (bowls, toys, flea collars), leather, motor oil, detergents, floor waxes, wool, synthetic rugs, fertilizers, insecticides, and mop sprays. Virtually any substance can cause sensitization in an individual.

CLINICAL PRESENTATION

Obviously, the lesions of irritant contact or allergic contact dermatitis are in the contact areas. The distribution of lesions will depend on the nature of the contactant. Reactions to topical medications occur at the site of application. Because animals can spread the medication by scratching or rubbing, lesions can occur around the area of application or on the foot used to scratch it. Medications applied to the whole body, such as shampoos or dips, will affect the whole body. Intertriginous areas, such as the axillary or inguinal regions or the skin between the pads, are usually most severely involved because these areas are moist and tend to accumulate materials that come in close contact with the skin.

Environmental contact sensitivities initially cause lesions in sparsely haired or hairless areas. The chin, feet, axillary and inguinal areas, tail, and perineum are usually involved (Figs. 8–1 and 8–2). Pedal involvement affects the skin around or between the pads but not the pads themselves. If the contactant is a substance on a flat smooth surface such as a floor wax, the skin between the pads may not be affected. Powders, liquids, or contactants on irregular surfaces, such as carpet fibers or plants, will affect the entire plantar surface of the paw and distal extremity. Animals with atopy usually have lesions on the dorsum of the paw, while those with contact dermatitis have disease of the ventral surface. The more chronic the allergy, the more widespread the eruption, since pruritus damages the skin and removes hair, which exposes new areas.

The clinical features of acute allergic contact dermatitis include erythema and swelling with variable pruritus. Papules or plaques may be seen if the self-trauma is not too severe. Bullae or vesicles are rare. As the dermatitis becomes more chronic, the skin becomes thickened, lichenified, crusted, and usually hyperpigmented. Secondary pyodermas and seborrheic changes can be superimposed on the contact dermatitis.

The features of allergic contact dermatitis are not distinctive; the differential diagnosis would include irritant contact dermatitis, atopy, food allergy, seborrheic dermatitis, scabies, hookworm dermatitis, and *Pelodera* dermatitis.

DIAGNOSTIC APPROACH

The diagnosis of allergic contact dermatitis is not a neat and orderly process involving first the history, next the physical, and then the diagnostic test results; rather it is a continuing interaction using information obtained at each of these steps.

The history can be of a seasonal or nonseasonal nature depending on the type of contactant. If many animals are involved or if the

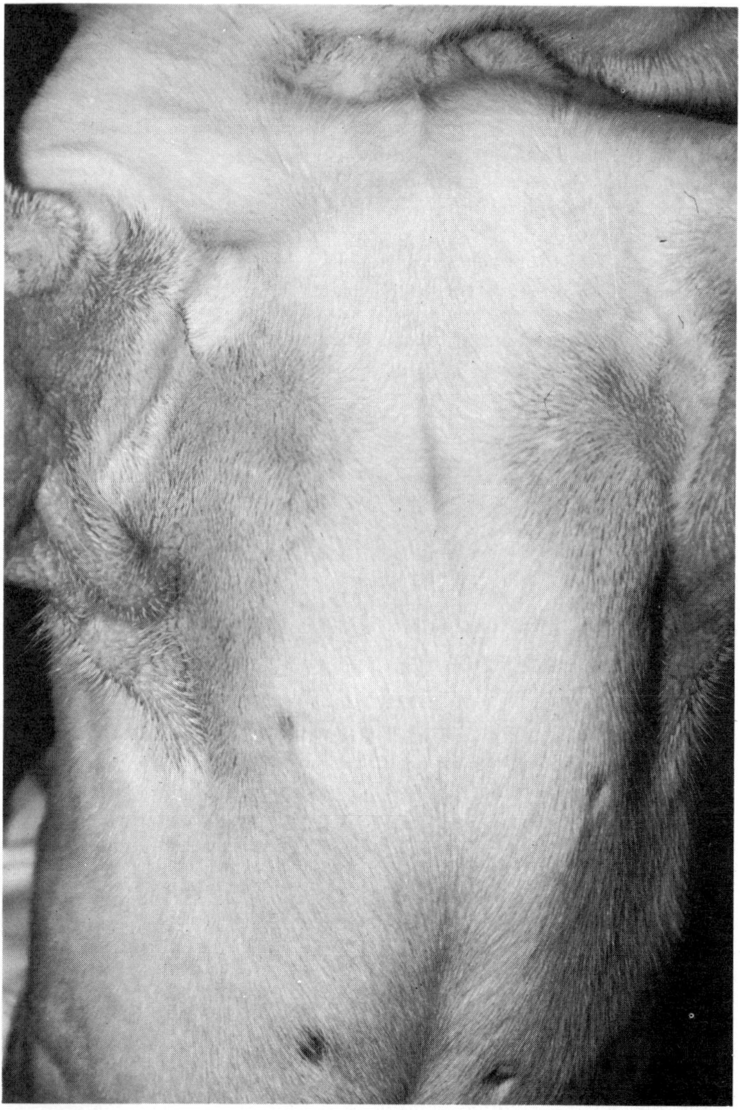

FIGURE 8–1. Alopecia, erythema, and lichenification of the axillary skin in a dog sensitive to a floor wax.

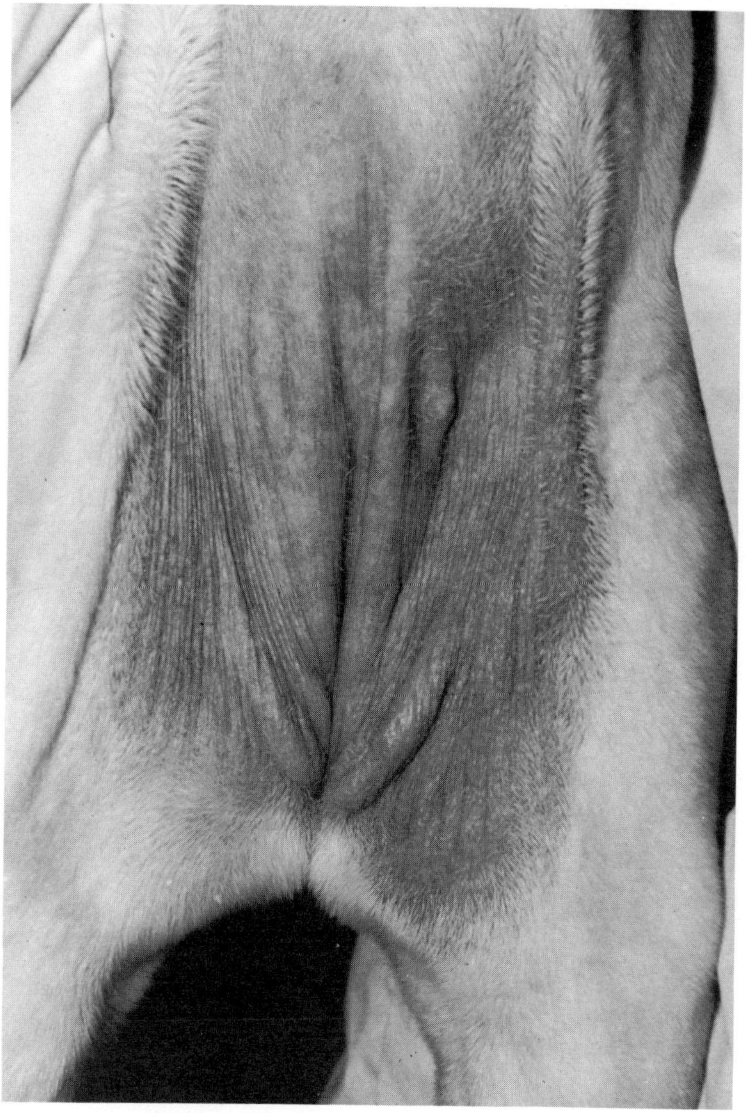

FIGURE 8–2. The ventral abdomen of the dog.

pruritus truly preceded the lesions, allergic contact dermatitis is very unlikely. If the history indicates that the problem started simultaneously with an environmental change, irritant dermatitis is more likely. It has been shown that approximately 70 percent of dogs with allergic contact dermatitis have been exposed to the offending substance for at least two years before developing clinical sensitivity. Accordingly, it would be unusual to see allergic contact dermatitis in the very young animal. After the physical examination and routine diagnostic tests are completed, one can often offer the tentative diagnosis of contact dermatitis. Additional historic information should then be sought to identify possible contactants.

Routine diagnostic tests should include skin scrapings for scabies, *Demodex* and *Pelodera*, a fecal examination for hookworms, and a fungal culture. Skin testing and hypoallergenic diets should be utilized as appropriate. Skin biopsies are helpful but nondiagnostic because superficial perivascular dermatitis with hyperplasia and spongiosis is usually seen. If epidermal necrosis is present, acute irritant dermatitis is most likely.

To confirm the diagnosis of contact dermatitis, isolation techniques or patch testing must be done, although isolation techniques do not distinguish between irritant contact and allergic contact dermatitis. True positive patch test results prove contact allergy.

Patch Testing

Patch tests are used to determine whether a patient has a type IV hypersensitivity to a specific substance. Suspect agents are placed in pure form on normal bare skin, and the test site is examined in 48 hours for signs of reaction. Reactions in animals are usually not very inflammatory and consist of erythema and edema.

In human medicine, standardized commercial patch test kits are available, which include common sensitizers at nonirritating concentrations. Such kits are not available in veterinary medicine, and the applicability of human kits to animals is unproven. Walton has suggested some concentrations and vehicles for patch testing dogs (Table 8–1).

Patch testing can be done in an open or closed fashion. Normal skin must be used for the testing and the animal must not be receiving anti-inflammatory medications. The back or lateral thorax is a common test site. The test site should be clipped several days before the test because clipper irritation can cause false-positive reactions. Trauma to the test site will invalidate the test, so an Elizabethan collar and foot bandages should be placed on the animal.

Closed Patch Testing

In closed patch testing, pure test materials are dissolved or suspended in an appropriate medium, usually petrolatum, and

TABLE 8–1. Suggested Concentrations and Vehicles for Canine Patch Testing

SUBSTANCE	CONCENTRATION AND VEHICLE
DYES	
Acetanilid, acridine, alizarin red 1034, aniline black, aniline brilliant green, anthraquinone, anthraquinone blue, chrome yellow	Powder
Alizarin red, hair dyes, naphthol yellow, nigrosin, Nile blue, pontamine black, rhodamine B, safranine, tartrazine blue, Victoria blue	Undiluted
Fuchsin, methylaniline, indigo	10% solution
Alizarin 778, methyl violet	2% solution
Aniline dyes	2% in olive oil or paraffin
Diazonium salts	1% in paraffin
Fluorescein	1% in 70% alcohol
MORDANTS AND INTERMEDIATES	
Chrome alum	Undiluted
Cobalt oxide, naphthalene	Undiluted
Chromium potassium sulfate, formaldehyde, naphthol	10% aqueous
Copper sulfate, pyrogallol, sodium thiosulfate	2% aqueous
Chromium chloride, chromium sulfate, picric acid	2% aqueous
Hydroxymercurichlorphenol, tannic acid	0.5% aqueous
MISCELLANEOUS	
Floor cleaners, detergents, dirt repellents, aluminum chloride	1% aqueous*
Nickel sulfate	5% aqueous
Floor polishes and waxes	5% in olive oil or 70% alcohol*
Medicaments	At therapeutic dose*
Oleoresins	As instructed
Dyed objects	Attempt to extract with water, alcohol, olive oil, acetone, chloroform

*If in doubt, or following a positive reaction, carry out control tests on normal animals to exclude possible irritant reactions. (From Walton, G.S. (ed): Current Veterinary Therapy VI. Philadelphia, W.B. Saunders Company, 1977, p. 575.)

applied to the skin. If pure test materials are unavailable, suspect agents such as carpet fibers, plant leaves, and waxes can be used. The test antigen is applied to pieces of filter paper, which are placed on the skin. The pieces of paper are held in place under a flexible, occlusive plastic tape, and the whole test site is covered with a bandage.

The bandage and test antigens are removed in 48 to 72 hours, and the test sites are marked. When the bandage is removed, the site will be reddened because of the occlusion of the bandage or the cleaning used to remove the excess antigens. This erythema will subside in 15 to 60 minutes, and then the test can be read. The sites should be examined by the owner for the next several days to see if any late reactions occur.

Open Patch Testing

With open patch testing, test materials suspended in the appropriate medium are simply rubbed on the skin, and the test sites are examined daily for five days. To prevent mixing of one test antigen into another, the test sites should be far apart. Thus, the number of tests should be kept small. The test site must be protected from water, dirt, self-trauma, and so forth.

Interpretation of Patch Test Results

All true positive reactions are significant, but they may not be clinically relevant. The reaction could indicate an old sensitivity or portend a future problem. The history must be examined to determine if the allergen is in the environment.

A more troublesome problem is a false-positive or a false-negative reaction. False-negative results may be due to the failure to include all the appropriate test antigens or to poor antigen penetration. Poor site occlusion, or protection, can affect penetration, as can the concentration of the antigens. Contactants, especially medications, are often applied to damaged skin. This skin is more permeable than normal skin used for testing. In the clinical situation, penetration can be enhanced by increasing the concentration of the test agent. For example, neomycin is usually tested at a 20 percent concentration even though the concentration in most medications is 0.5 percent.

False-positive results can occur because the test agents were too concentrated and therefore were irritating, or because the test was done on diseased skin. Careful site selection should eliminate the latter problem. Since patch test kits are not standardized in veterinary medicine, the possibility of irritation always exists. Any positive reactant should ideally be tested on a normal animal to see if it is irritating.

Isolation Techniques

With all the problems associated with patch testing, it is not very commonly used. Isolation techniques can support the diagnosis of a contact dermatitis, and if the owners are very dedicated, the offending substance can be identified.

The animal should be removed from the suspected agent or environment for 7 to 10 days. Prior to removal, the animal should be bathed with a hypoallergenic shampoo to remove residual contactants from the skin. If the animal improves with avoidance, the diagnosis of allergic contact dermatitis is supported but not proven. Provocative exposure testing is necessary. If the signs recur upon re-exposure, the diagnosis is confirmed and the etiologic agent(s) has been identified.

If the suspect contactant is something simple such as a food bowl or toy, the isolation procedure is straightforward. If an environmental agent is involved, the whole procedure becomes much more complicated. If the dog is normal during its stay in a kennel, and if the signs recur when it is returned to its normal environment, a great deal of detective work will be necessary. A nonallergenic environment must be found (kennel, child's play pen, basement) and the animal must be kept there. Suspect agents such as carpets or floor cleaners are placed in the "clean" room in sufficient quantity that the animal will touch them. If a reaction is seen immediately, the animal has an irritant dermatitis. Allergic reactions should not take place for several days. If a reaction occurs, the substance is removed and the animal is immediately bathed. If the history suggests multiple sensitivities, the testing should be continued once the skin has returned to normal. Obviously this type of testing requires a very dedicated owner and a cooperative pet.

TREATMENT

Avoidance is curative; however, this requires the identification of the causative agent. If this is possible, the dermatitis will resolve spontaneously in 7 to 14 days. Bathing to remove the residual contactant will hasten the response, and glucocorticoids can be used to lessen the pruritus and inflammation.

More typically, the offending agent cannot be identified or cannot be removed. In this instance, symptomatic steroid therapy will be necessary. Anti-inflammatory levels of steroids are used daily for 7 to 14 days, and then they are administered on alternate days or less frequently. Frequent bathing can decrease the animal's allergen load and lower the dose of steroids.

Immunotherapy is of little or no value in allergic contact dermatitis.

9 Fleas and Flea Bite Hypersensitivity

INTRODUCTION

Fleas are insect parasites of dogs, cats, pigs, rodents, rabbits, birds, and humans. In addition to being annoying, fleas can be vectors for various diseases and can produce allergic reactions in some individuals.

Fleas are the most common external parasite of companion animals and are an important cause of skin disease. In the southern part of the United States, fleas are believed to be a major factor in more than 50 percent of small animal dermatology cases.

ANATOMY AND LIFE CYCLE

Fleas (order Siphonaptera) are small wingless insects with laterally compressed bodies and a thick, brown chitinous covering. Powerful legs adapted for jumping enable fleas to readily transfer from host to host. There are approximately 1500 species of fleas, although *Ctenocephalides felis*, *Ctenocephalides canis*, and *Pulex irritans* are the most common species that infest the dog and cat. Halliwell believes that *C. canis* is fast becoming extinct.

In the adult stage, all fleas are blood-sucking ectoparasites of warm-blooded animals. Most flea species, especially when hungry, show limited host specificity. During feeding, specialized mouthparts pierce the host's skin to siphon blood. Saliva is injected into the wound to prevent the blood from clotting. Adult fleas can live for long periods without feeding, but a blood meal is necessary for reproduction.

Fleas develop by complete metamorphosis. Copulation occurs after a blood meal, and the female can lay up to 20 eggs at one time. The eggs are small, ovoid, white, and nonsticky. Eggs can be laid in the environment or on the host, but as the eggs are not adherent, most of the eggs fall off into the environment. The number of eggs laid as well as the development rate of the flea is temperature- and humidity-dependent. The female can lay 400 to 500 eggs in its lifetime.

There are three larval stages called instars. The larvae are very active and try to avoid light. They are creamy yellow in color, legless, and maggot-like with masticating mouthparts and two posterior hooked parts called anal struts. The struts are used for locomotion, grasping, and holding. Very little food is necessary for development, but the larvae do ingest organic matter, especially blood-containing feces that fall from the host. Shortly after molting, the third instar spins an oval, sticky cocoon in which it pupates to form the adult. The eggs and cocoons are very resistant to weather conditions, insecticides, and chemicals.

The rate of development depends greatly on temperature and humidity (Fig. 9–1). Although the general weather in an area may be hot and dry, the climatic conditions where fleas and their larvae hide may be significantly different. Under optimal conditions of a moderate temperature (65 to 80° F) and high humidity (70 percent), the life cycle can be completed in as short as 14 days. At low (55° F) or high (90° F) temperatures, the life cycle can take up to 140 days. Temperatures above 90° F are lethal to larvae and pupae, and hard rains can drown them.

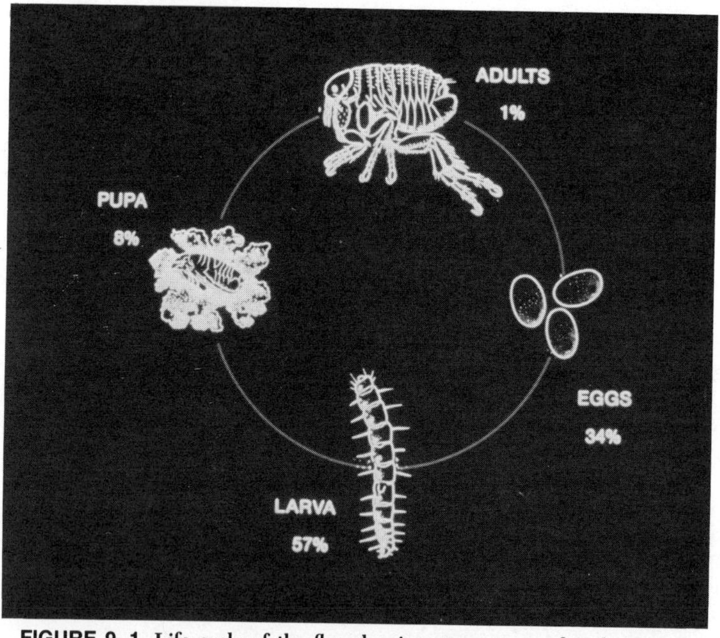

FIGURE 9–1. Life cycle of the flea showing percentages of each stage at any given time. (Courtesy of L. Veith, VetKem.)

Adult fleas are very hardy, and when feeding, they can survive for long periods in unfavorable conditions. Unfed adults do not live long in dry or subfreezing conditions. In the laboratory, *C. felis*, the most common flea, survives for 234 days if it is unfed. Under more natural conditions, it has been estimated that *C. canis* can live for 26 months.

HOST DISTRIBUTION

While the common names for fleas (dog flea, cat flea, and so on) might imply some host specificity, no such specificity exists. Hungry fleas will feed from almost any warm-blooded animal. The cat flea (*C. felis*), the dog flea (*C. canis*), and the human flea (*P. irritans*) are the most problematic to pets, but the poultry or sticktight flea (*Echidnophaga gallinacea*), the rat flea (*Xenopsylla cheopis*), the mouse flea (*Leptopsylla segnis*), and the chigoe flea (*Tunga penetrans*) also cause problems. The saliva of *C. felis*, *P. irritans*, and *P. simulans* share common antigens. If an animal is hypersensitive to the bite of one species of flea, it probably will show hypersensitivity to the bites of other species.

Flea saliva contains histamine-like compounds and enzymes that are proteolytic, anticoagulant, and cytolytic in nature and have hyaluronidase-like activity. Since these substances are injected into the host during feeding, the flea bite is irritating. The poultry flea and the chigoe or sand flea burrow into the host's skin and cause severe irritation. As mentioned before, flea saliva is antigenic as well as irritating, so both flea bite dermatitis and flea bite hypersensitivity have been noted.

FLEA BITE DERMATITIS

Flea bite dermatitis is a nonallergic condition caused by the irritation of the flea bite. Most pets will do some chewing or scratching when bitten by fleas. Clinically significant flea bite dermatitis is much less common than flea allergy dermatitis.

The clinical sign of flea bite dermatitis is a pruritic papular eruption. In the dog, common areas of involvement include the lower back, tail, posterior and medial thighs, and the inguinal region. In the cat, crusted papules are found between the shoulder blades and along the lower back. The severity of the clinical signs is usually related to the number of flea bites. Some nervous pets or those with very sensitive skin will scratch out of proportion to the number of flea bites and will appear to be flea allergic.

The diagnosis of flea bite dermatitis is made by physical examination and demonstration of fleas or flea excreta. A skin test with flea antigen should show no immediate or delayed reaction.

FLEA BITE HYPERSENSITIVITY

Flea bite hypersensitivity is a pruritic, papular, crusted dermatitis in animals that have become sensitized to antigenic material in flea saliva. Flea bite hypersensitivity, also called flea allergy dermatitis, is the most common allergic skin disease of the dog and cat. The incidence is unknown but probably varies with the climate and flea population.

The distinction between nonallergic flea bite dermatitis and flea bite hypersensitivity can sometimes be difficult. In nonallergic flea bite dermatitis, there usually is a direct relationship between the number of flea bites and the degree of reaction. In pets with very sensitive skin, i.e., those that are atopic or flea allergic, this relationship does not always exist. In very allergic patients, a few flea bites can produce a severe allergic reaction.

Pathogenesis

The pathogenesis of flea bite hypersensitivity has been extensively studied in the guinea pig and is currently being studied in the dog. Flea saliva contains histamine-like compounds, enzymes, polypeptides, amino acids, aromatic compounds, and fluorescent materials. Gel filtration of flea saliva reveals that allergens are present in a high molecular weight fraction (4000 to 10,000 daltons) and in a highly fluorescent aromatic fraction (less than 1000 daltons). In the guinea pig, intradermal or intraperitoneal injection of flea saliva failed to cause sensitization. Coupling the saliva with an adjuvant caused sensitization, thus indicating that the allergen was a low molecular weight simple chemical, or hapten. Dermal collagen appeared to be the cutaneous adjuvant for the hapten. In view of our knowledge of immunology and flea bite hypersensitivity in the dog, other complete allergens must also be present in flea saliva. A flea bite or an intradermal injection of flea antigen will usually cause an immediate wheal reaction, which is thought to be IgE-mediated. This type of hypersensitivity reaction requires the bridging of two adjacent mast cell–bound IgE molecules, which cannot be accomplished by a univalent hapten. In the dog, a major allergen in flea saliva appears to be a protein of a molecular weight between 5000 and 10,000 daltons. Other components may also be allergenic.

In the guinea pig, an orderly process of sensitization and desensitization has been described. An asymptomatic induction period is followed by stage II in which the animals show predominantly delayed hypersensitivity reactions. Stage III shows concurrent immediate and delayed reactions. In stage IV, the delayed sensitivity is lost, while the immediate sensitivity persists. Finally, in stage V, all reactivity is lost within 20 weeks.

Recent studies have shown that this orderly process does not occur in the dog. In many instances, delayed reactions preceded the development of immediate reactions, although delayed reactions have been documented as occurring at the same time or even after the onset of immediate reactions. In general, most flea-allergic dogs have both immediate and delayed skin test reactivity; 5 to 10 percent will show only an immediate or a delayed reaction. Delayed reactions can occur at 4 to 8 hours, 24 hours, or 48 hours.

In studies on the pathogenesis of flea allergy in the dog, Halliwell showed that dogs periodically exposed to fleas would develop positive skin tests in 2 to 12 weeks, while those constantly exposed to fleas developed their reactions much later and to a lesser extent. The episodically exposed animals typically had detectable levels of IgE and high levels of IgG against flea antigen, while the continuously exposed dogs had little detectable antibody of either class. These data suggest that continuous exposure can lead to a state of partial or complete immunologic tolerance. When the constantly exposed dogs were switched to an intermittent exposure, they developed skin test reactivity and IgE and IgG antibody responses, which suggests that they lost their tolerance. Once a dog developed reactivity, it persisted for the length of the study (44 weeks) rather than being lost early, as in the guinea pig.

Type I and type IV hypersensitivity reactions have been documented in the dog, but the variable histologic picture and the fact that delayed reactions can occur anywhere from 4 to 48 hours suggest the presence of another immunologic mechanism. A late-onset IgE reaction and cutaneous basophil hypersensitivity have been proposed as contributory immunologic mechanisms.

Cutaneous basophil hypersensitivity (Jones-Mote reaction) is a poorly understood type of delayed hypersensitivity with a predominantly basophil infiltration that occurs transiently within 24 hours after cutaneous rechallenge with sensitizing antigen. Cutaneous basophil hypersensitivity is a protective response in tick bite reactions. Antigen-specific IgE molecules bind to the receptors on the surface of basophils. These basophils are attracted to the site of a tick bite, and when the basophil comes in contact with the salivary antigens, the basophil degranulates. Histamine is the primary effector substance released from the basophil, which mediates the death of the tick.

In a study on cutaneous basophil hypersensitivity in canine flea allergy, the number of basophils at the site of an intradermal injection of flea antigen increased from 4 to 18 hours after the injection. The peak occurred at 12 hours, and the number had substantially fallen by 48 hours. Mononuclear cells increased after 18 hours, while the percentage of eosinophils was fairly constant. These data support the contention that cutaneous basophil hypersensitivity may play a role in the immunopathogenesis of flea bite hypersensitivity.

Since fleas usually do not stay attached to the skin for long periods of time, cutaneous basophil hypersensitivity may be more detrimental than protective in flea allergy. Some degree of protection is suggested by the fact that flea hypersensitive dogs have fewer female fleas on their bodies than do other dogs. Female fleas spend more time on the dog's body than do male fleas and therefore are more likely to be killed by the cutaneous basophil hypersensitivity. The poultry flea (*E. gallinacea*) and the sand flea (*T. penetrans*) are burrowing fleas and would be more susceptible to the effects of basophil hypersensitivity. The detrimental effect of cutaneous basophil hypersensitivity revolves around the persistence of the antigen at the site of the flea bite. The basophil will degranulate and release its vasoactive substances, causing inflammation of the skin without killing the flea, since it has already gone.

Clinical Features

There is no apparent breed or sex predilection for flea bite hypersensitivity. Interestingly, in atopic dogs, the incidence of positive skin tests to flea antigen has been reported to be approximately 80 percent as compared with a 40 percent incidence in the general population. This suggests that the atopic state favors the development or the maintenance of the flea allergic state. Accordingly, those breeds prone to atopy would be more likely to develop flea bite hypersensitivity. Flea bite hypersensitivity can develop at any age, but it is rare in animals less than six months of age. The most common age of onset is three to six years.

In those parts of the country where there is a flea season, flea bite hypersensitivity is a seasonal disorder with peak incidence during the late summer and early fall. Chronically allergic animals will start to scratch earlier and will show signs into winter. Provided that the house is not infested, the signs should resolve in the dead of winter. In warm parts of the country or in infested houses, flea allergy can be a nonseasonal problem with seasonal variations.

The signs of flea bite hypersensitivity are similar to those of nonallergic flea bite dermatitis but are much more profound. The intensity of the signs does not correlate with the number of fleas found. The primary lesion in both the dog and cat is a papule that may develop a significant surrounding area of erythema. The papules usually become crusted. Lesions will be found anywhere the flea feeds. In the dog, the lower back, tail, posterior and medial thighs, and ventrum are primarily affected, while the cat often has additional lesions between the shoulder blades. Because of the allergic nature of this condition, the primary lesions are often confused or masked by signs of self-trauma. In the dog, acute moist dermatitis, secondary pyoderma, alopecia, and secondary seborrhea are common findings. In the cat, severe excoriations, eosinophilic plaques, or linear granulomas can be superimposed on the underlying miliary dermatitis.

In severely allergic animals, a generalized cutaneous reaction may occur. The flea hypersensitivity of some severely affected dogs clinically resembles sarcoptic mange. In some cases, the owners will complain of facial and pedal pruritus in their animals, which coexist with rump itching. This atopic-type pruritus can be explained by flea bites in those areas, concurrent atopy or food allergy, or a generalized IgE-mediated flea hypersensitivity.

DIAGNOSIS

A diagnosis of flea bite hypersensitivity can be proposed based on the physical findings. Demonstration of fleas or flea excreta supports but does not confirm the diagnosis, as the fleas may be a coincidental finding. Alternatively, flea hypersensitivity can exist without direct evidence of fleas. Elimination of the clinical signs with the eradication of the flea supports the diagnosis but does not prove the hypersensitivity because immunologic abnormalities have not been documented.

In the dog and cat, the differential diagnoses include atopy, food hypersensitivity, folliculitis, drug hypersensitivity, and intestinal parasite hypersensitivity. In the cat, the most common cause of miliary dermatitis is flea allergy, but all other causes of this disease, such as *Cheyletiella* infestation, atopy, food allergy, and dermatophytosis, must also be considered.

In most cases, the clinical signs coupled with the presence of fleas are sufficient for diagnosis. Although the clinician may find fleas on the animal, the owner often cannot. A flea comb is an excellent clinical aid allowing the fleas or flea excreta to be removed from the animal and shown to the owner. The owner should be shown how to identify flea excreta, as this may be the only indication of the presence of fleas once flea control is started. A moistened white paper towel will turn reddish-brown around specks of "dirt" if the material is flea excreta. Street dirt will not cause the color change, but bloody crusts from skin wounds will. Bloody crusts are larger than flea excreta and the color change takes longer.

Skin biopsies can show a superficial perivascular dermatitis typical of allergic disease. If eosinophils are the prominent dermal cell type or if eosinophilic intraepidermal microabscesses are seen, flea bite hypersensitivity is strongly suggested, although these features may not be seen. Hemograms may or may not show a peripheral eosinophilia.

Intradermal skin testing with flea antigen has been advocated as the diagnostic test for flea bite hypersensitivity. Unfortunately, the results of the skin test are not foolproof. Negative reactions do not exclude the diagnosis, while true positive results indicate a sensitivity that may or may not be the cause of the animal's problem. Figures indicating the sensitivity and specificity of flea antigen skin testing vary greatly. Van Winkle states that commercial flea antigens are not satisfactory for testing, while Halliwell reports that 98 percent of dogs with flea allergy show positive skin test. One author (LMR) tested 193 dogs suspected of being flea allergic, and only 45 percent reacted immediately to the flea antigen.

The questionable reliability of flea antigen for diagnostic purposes probably relates to the quality of the products available. Most products are whole flea extracts so that the concentration of the true allergen(s) is very low. Products containing glycerin are irritant and are very unreliable, while aqueous extracts tend to be less irritating. However, aqueous products can be irritating if used at concentrations greater than 1:1000. Another point of difficulty relates to the times at which the skin test is read. Halliwell reports that approximately 80 percent of skin test–positive dogs show immediate reactions; 10 percent show only delayed reactions; the remainder exhibit both. Flea skin tests should be read at 15 to 30 minutes, at 4 to 8 hours (cutaneous basophil hypersensitivity), and at 24 and 48 hours (delayed hypersensitivity reaction). Often it is impractical for the veterinarian to read other than the immediate test results. Owners are asked to read the sites for the delayed reactions, but these reports can be erroneous.

Presently, intradermal skin testing with flea antigen should be considered a supportive but not absolutely diagnostic test. Aqueous, nonglycerinated extracts should be used at a concentration of no greater than 1:1000 (W/V) and should be injected with appropriate positive and negative controls. The test should be read at the times previously mentioned. Animals that show delayed reactions will usually react at 24 hours rather than at 48 hours, and the reaction often will be an erythematous papule or plaque rather than the classic wheal. Skin testing can be very detrimental when dealing with a very skeptical client. A positive result may sway the client into believing the diagnosis, while a negative result may negate any further discussion or therapy for flea allergy. In these cases, it probably is best not to test only for fleas.

TREATMENT

Flea bite hypersensitivity can be treated by those methods used for the atopic animal—avoidance, immunotherapy, and medical management. Avoidance is the ideal treatment for nonallergic or allergic flea bite dermatitis and is discussed under clinical management. Steroidal or nonsteroidal anti-inflammatory drugs will usually be necessary when the animal is first presented. Chronic medical management without attempts at flea control will be unrewarding and should be discouraged. Since the flea is such a persistent parasite, some patients will need continued medical therapy, although intense flea control should lessen the allergenic load, thus decreasing the level of drugs needed.

Immunotherapy

The efficacy of immunotherapy for flea bite hypersensitivity is extremely controversial. Some clinical reports extol its virtues; others do not substantiate the findings. Two double-blind studies at the University of Florida concluded that the flea antigen injections currently available cannot be recommended for therapy. Halliwell studied the response of flea-allergic dogs to six weekly intradermal injections of various commercial flea antigens, while Kunkle studied the response of cats to 20 weekly intradermal or subcutaneous injections of one particular antigen. Kunkle found that 2 of her 18 treated cats responded markedly, while one additional cat showed moderate improvement. One of the cats that showed marked improvement received intradermal injections; the other received subcutaneous injections. The cat that improved moderately also received subcutaneous injections. In Halliwell's study, some improvement was noted in some of the dogs, but the overall assessment was that his protocol probably was not helpful.

The apparent ineffectiveness of flea immunotherapy in animals agrees with similar studies in humans with insect hypersensitivity. However, in humans, it has been shown that immunotherapy with insect venom is much more efficacious than using whole insect extracts. A better flea antigen would probably increase the efficacy of immunotherapy in pets.

Presently, immunotherapy for flea allergy cannot be recommended except as a last step before euthanasia or chronic steroid management. If immunotherapy is attempted, it should be used in conjunction with the best flea control program attainable. Weekly intradermal injections of 0.5 to 1.0 ml of a commercial flea antigen should be given for 6 to 12 weeks or longer. The injections should be given at multiple sites over the back. If a response is seen, the vaccine should be given as needed prior to and during flea season. If no response is seen after 12 injections, it is unlikely that continued immunotherapy will be helpful.

Clinical Management

In general, flea bite hypersensitivity is a progressive disease. Each year, clinical signs begin earlier in the season, are more severe, and persist longer, making clinical management more difficult. The cure for this disorder is complete eradication of the flea from the patient and its environment. Unfortunately, this is extremely difficult if not impossible in some areas.

Until an effective method of immunotherapy becomes available, medical management will be necessary. Initially, animals with a flea bite hypersensitivity respond well to corticosteroid therapy even if no flea control program is instituted. As the animal becomes more hypersensitive or the flea burden increases, the response to glucocorticoid therapy decreases. A well-designed flea control program is the key factor in the management of flea bite hypersensitivity.

The control of fleas requires a well-organized comprehensive program that the client can understand. The owner must understand the hypersensitivity phenomenon and the nature of the flea and its life cycle. Most clients cannot absorb all of the necessary information in one short office visit, and thus lapses in control can be expected. Some written information given to the client is an excellent management tool. The handout should explain the life cycle of the flea and should describe in general terms the methods of flea control for the pet, for other household pets, and in the environment. A separate sheet should be attached with specific instructions for the products to be used for the individual client. The client can read and absorb the information at leisure and refer back to the document as needed, since flea control is an ongoing battle.

In those parts of the country where there is a flea season, every effort should be made to eradicate the fleas from the environment during the winter. Once this is done, the animal should be normal until the next flea season. An owner with a flea-allergic pet should start flea control in the early spring, even if the animal's problem does not historically start until summer. The institution of early treatment will emphasize the necessity of good flea control and usually will prevent or minimize the infestation of the pet's environment. If environmental infestation can be prevented, the management of the pet's hypersensitivity will be much easier and more rewarding.

FLEA CONTROL

An animal can be infested by fleas from its environment or by contact with other animals. Intense treatment of a flea-allergic pet, which concentrates on the affected animal but ignores other household pets and the environment, will be unrewarding. A well-organized program should be designed for the specific situation in question and should include the treatment of the environment as well as all animals. Environmental management is the most difficult and expensive part of the program but is the key to success.

Since flea problems are so widespread, and since millions of dollars are spent annually on flea control products, new or upgraded insecticides and their delivery systems are constantly being introduced. Although many factors enter into the selection of an insecticide and its delivery system, the residual and repellent effect of the product should be of paramount importance. Unfortunately, the data collected from the laboratory often do not apply to the clinical situation.

Treatment of Animals

Unfortunately, electronic flea collars and dietary supplements of brewer's yeast, garlic, elemental sulfur, and so forth are ineffective in the control of fleas. These remedies may lessen the flea burden but do not eradicate fleas. Insecticides must be used. Commonly used insecticides include botanic products (pyrethrins, rotenone, and *d*-limonene), synthetic pyrethroids, organophosphates, and carbamates. These insecticides can be applied via a flea collar, shampoo, aerosol spray, pump spray, foam, dust, dip, or pour-on. One organophosphate, Proban, is approved for oral administration in the dog.

The selection of the insecticide depends on the local resistance of the flea population, the species of animal being treated, the coat quality of the animal, and the wishes of the owner. Some owners will not use toxic chemicals on their pets, and thus the veterinarian is restricted to the use of botanic products. Fleas can become resistant to insecticides and any local resistance must be considered. In many instances, "resistance" is actually due to poor application technique rather than true biochemical resistance. Most insecticides will kill fleas, but environmental infestation or the short residual effect of the applied product is such that fleas will quickly reinfest the animal.

One should select insecticides that are approved for use on both dogs and cats of all ages and are not too stringent in their labeling directions. Products labeled for use no more frequently than once every two to three weeks give the veterinarian very little flexibility. In the clinical situation, few if any insecticides will be fully effective for three weeks. More frequent application of these potent products may be toxic to the animal and is an "extra-label" use of the product. The best products to use are those that are labeled without interval restrictions or can be modified by the direction of the veterinarian. With these products, the insecticide can be used safely and legally as needed.

The method of application depends on the nature of the animal, the local weather conditions, and the owner's wishes. Cats often resent liquid products leaving the choice among flea collars, powders, and foams. If the owner and animal will tolerate any method of application, the size of the pet and the nature of its coat dictate the appropriate method. Flea shampoos have little or no residual effect and thus are a poor choice as a sole means of flea control. Flea dusts or powders may not be effective in animals with short coats, such as the dachshund, since the powder will fall from the body when the dog shakes. Alternatively, dogs with dense undercoats, such as the chow chow, are poor candidates for powders, aerosol sprays, pump sprays, and foams because these products are difficult to apply to the skin. Pressurized aerosol sprays have little applicability in most animals since pets resent and resist their application. Pump sprays and foams have the greatest applicability in animals with short to normal coats. Since these products are more expensive than flea dips, they are used most economically in small animals. Flea misting a large, long-haired dog such as a golden retriever would take a long time and a large volume of flea mist.

Flea dips are the most thorough method to apply an insecticide, but they are also the messiest. In warm weather, dogs can be dipped outside, but during cold or rainy weather, many owners are reluctant to dip their large pets. Small- to medium-sized dogs can be done in a bath tub, but large dogs can be a problem. In this case, the dip can be applied by a pump spray. The owner should buy a pump bottle and mix enough dip solution to fill the reservoir. Unless the flea dip is stable after dilution, the unused portion should be discarded. Self-mixed mists require significant application time for large dogs, but they are considerably less expensive than commercial products, and they leave the animal damp but not soaking wet.

For animals that swim frequently or that will not tolerate sprays, powders, foams, and dips, flea collars or systemic organophosphates are the only other alternatives. The two approved systemic organophosphates for dogs are Pro-Spot and Proban. Proban is administered orally twice weekly; Pro-Spot is applied to the skin every two weeks. Spot-On is a cattle insecticide similar but not identical to Pro-Spot. Both products contain fenthion, which is rapidly absorbed after dermal application, but Spot-On is not approved for use in pets. With these products, the flea ingests a lethal dose of the insecticide while it is feeding on the animal. Some veterinarians believe that Spot-On has some repellent activity as well.

The most important aspect of flea control on animals is not the quick killing of the flea but rather the residual effectiveness of the product(s). Many product brochures claim a residual time that is not substantiated in the clinical situation. This discrepancy could be explained by poor owner application, environmental infestation, or animal habits such as swimming or grooming. An effective, well-applied standard flea dip will appear to be effective only for 12 to 24 hours if the animal's environment is heavily infested. Current technologic advances that have increased the residual effectiveness of flea products include the development of the synthetic pyrethroids and the microencapsulation technology. However, no topical product will be solely effective in a heavily infested environment.

Since many animal and environmental flea products contain organophosphates or carbamates, care must be taken not to poison the animal. Carbamates should not be used on animals treated with organophosphates and vice versa. Pyrethrins and pyrethroids can be used in conjunction with either organophosphates or carbamates.

Treatment of the Flea Hypersensitive Animal

In the flea-allergic animal, the goal of therapy is to prevent all flea bites. Flea shampoos, flea collars, casual flea dips, and the currently approved systemic organophosphates are inadequate as the sole means of flea control. Intense topical insecticidal therapy is necessary.

Carbamate flea powders (5 percent) applied two to three times weekly are effective for cats and partially effective for dogs. Dogs are sparsely haired along the ventrum, and thus the powder has poor holding power. Pump sprays (containing carbamates, pyrethrins, or pyrethroids) can be used on the ventrum to increase the efficacy of the powder. Intense powdering will dry the animal's coat because of the absorptive nature of the talc base.

Pump sprays are very effective for both dogs and cats provided the coat allows penetration of the mist. Most mists contain synergized pyrethrins in either an alcohol or aqueous base. Alcohol-based products have a more rapid kill rate but can dry or irritate the skin especially if it is already inflamed. The pyrethrin sprays can be used daily. Pyrethroid sprays or those that contain microencapsulated pyrethrins are more expensive, but they have a longer residual effect and need only be used once or twice weekly. Pump sprays that contain organophosphates or carbamates should be used every fourth to seventh day as the label directs. If fleas are seen before the next application, it probably would be best to switch to a pyrethrin or pyrethroid product.

Innumerable flea dips are marketed. The frequency of application depends on the toxicity of the product. Organophosphate and carbamate dips should be applied no more frequently than every fifth day. In peak flea season, fleas will usually be seen on the animal before the next application. Pyrethrin/pyrethroid pump sprays can be used to supplement the dip, or a pyrethrin/pyrethroid dip can be used. Frequent dipping will dry the animal's coat. The addition of a bath oil or humectant to the diluted flea dip will help minimize the drying.

In those situations in which the flea-allergic dog swims daily or its owner will not use intense topical therapy, systemic organophosphate products have some applicability. Unless the unlicensed product Spot-On is used, or Pro-Spot or Proban is used in an "extra-labeled" fashion, complete control will not be achieved. Pyrethrin/pyrethroid sprays or dips can be safely used to supplement the effect of the systemic product. Although these systemic organophosphates have been used on cats, they are not approved for use in this species.

Treatment of Contact Animals

Ideally, all contact dogs and cats should be treated with as much vigor as the flea-hypersensitive pet. If the client owns many animals, especially cats, the cost and time commitment of this intense therapy may be prohibitive. Systemic organophosphates can be used to treat the dogs, while flea collars will help decrease the flea population on the cats.

Treatment of the Environment

Environmental management is the most crucial part of any flea control program. None of the products used on animals is 100 percent effective, so intense animal treatment alone is almost a waste of time and money if the environment is heavily infested. Environmental management is expensive and time-consuming, so prevention of infestation is the primary goal. In those parts of the country where there is a flea season, every effort should be made to eradicate the flea from the house, kennel, or barn during the winter. In early spring, flea control should be started on the animals. The aim of this early therapy is to prevent the animals from bringing fleas into the house or kennel. If the indoor flea burden is minimized, the pets should have few or no problems.

INDOOR FLEA CONTROL

Ultrasonic insect repellent devices, boric acid, and other home remedies have little effect on the indoor flea population. Cleaning and insecticidal therapy must be used. It must be emphasized to the owners that they have to eliminate the adult fleas as well as the eggs, larvae, and pupae.

Eggs, larvae, pupae, and adult fleas will be found anywhere an animal rests. If the animal is restricted from certain rooms, these rooms should be flea-free. All other areas should be treated. Adult fleas will hide in cracks and crevices, between carpet fibers, under furniture, and under organic debris in the kennel. Immature forms will also be found in these areas. Insecticides penetrate poorly into some of these areas unless they are cleaned first.

Vacuuming is the first line of defense in the cleaning process. The carpets, furniture, areas under cushions, cracks in the floor, and the crevice along baseboards should be vacuumed carefully to remove as many of the immature flea forms as possible. Adults will usually not be caught by the vacuum. The vacuum bag should be discarded after the cleaning is complete; otherwise adult fleas can develop in and escape from the vacuum. Alternatively, mothballs can be put in the bag to kill fleas. Deep pile or shag carpets are very difficult to depopulate because vacuuming often does not remove the immature flea forms deep down in the carpet, and insecticides remain on the surface. Steam cleaning will be necessary to rid these carpets of fleas. Temperatures above 95° F are lethal to larvae and pupae. Kennels should be cleaned as carefully as the house. After the thorough cleaning, insecticides are applied to the house or kennel. Unless the insecticide literature suggests otherwise, the house or kennel should not be vacuumed for two weeks after the application as this can decrease the residual effectiveness.

A wide variety of insecticides are available through veterinarians, hardware stores, and exterminators. Products that contain only a quick-kill insecticide are cost-ineffective, as the immature forms will mature and repopulate the house very quickly. Insecticide products that combine a quick-kill agent with a growth regulator or a residual insecticide are preferred.

Many clients, especially those with young children, are averse to the idea of applying potent residual insecticides. Microencapsulation technology minimizes these concerns. A thin chemical shell covers a minute amount of the insecticide, protecting it and allowing its slow, sustained release. Microencapsulation protects pyrethrins from inactivation by ultraviolet light and significantly decreases the acute mammalian toxicity. This technology is being extended to more potent organophosphate insecticides.

Methoprene is a chemical that mimics insect growth hormone. Growth hormone is necessary for early larval growth and development, but decreased levels are necessary to trigger larval metamorphosis at the pupal stage. Sustained high levels of growth hormone, either natural or man-made, interrupt the maturation process, prevent pupation and, ultimately, result in larval death. Adults and pupae are not affected. Methoprene is light-sensitive and is ineffective in bright areas inside as well as outside.

It is difficult if not impossible to kill all of the adult fleas with one application of an insecticidal product. If a quick-kill plus residual insecticide product is used, any adults that are missed or that develop from immature forms will be killed during the effective period of the insecticide. With long or continuous flea seasons, the product will have to be applied many times. When a product containing a quick-kill insecticide plus methoprene is used, some adult fleas will probably be left in the environment. These adults are those that were missed by the "adulticides" or that have developed from already pupated larvae. Eggs laid by these fleas should not develop because of the methoprene, but the fleas themselves may cause problems for the animals in the house. The application of a quick-kill insecticide alone two to three weeks after the initial treatment should exterminate this residual adult population.

The key to effective environmental treatment is the delivery system. The best insecticide is of little use if it is applied poorly. An incomplete understanding of the flea habits and life cycle, coupled with misconceptions on how products work, have led to much wasted effort on the client's part. The most poorly understood delivery system is the fogger or bomb.

Foggers contain insecticides that are aerosolized into droplets. The droplets remain suspended in the air for some time and then fall to the ground by gravity where they dry on contact. The nozzle design and pressure system determines droplet size and, consequently, the dispersal of the insecticide. Large droplets fall to the ground relatively quickly, while fine particles stay suspended longer and can travel farther.

Foggers do not cover room corners well and do not penetrate to any great extent under furniture cushions or furniture. These areas tend to be where the flea infestation is heaviest. The droplets dry on contact and do not penetrate into carpets. A good surface coating, however, should kill many larvae and fleas. The package information of many foggers indicates that they cover between 4000 and 10,000 cubic feet. Since many houses have rooms smaller than that, clients often think that the insecticide will spread effectively to adjacent rooms. Doorways and corridors interfere with dispersal and limit the effective spread of the insecticide. All of these factors make foggers less effective than owners and veterinarians would like.

To make better use of the fogger technology, a separate bomb should be set off in each room, and the furniture should be moved before the fogger is started. If the furniture is moved into areas that normally bear traffic, the insecticide will cover the hidden areas (which typically are most infested). Corners and baseboards should be sprayed by hand before the fogger is started. Depending on the ingredients in the fogger, this procedure may have to be repeated in two to three weeks.

Many clients will not use foggers because they do not like the idea of an insecticide on their furniture, electronic equipment, and so forth. Sprays are appropriate in this case because the insecticide can be directed to the infested areas. Environmental insecticides are sold in aerosol cans, pump sprays, and as concentrates. Aerosol sprays are most convenient but are expensive and difficult to direct under furniture. Pump sprays are more economical but can cause hand fatigue, especially if large areas need to be sprayed. For the owner who is serious about spraying large areas, a compressed air or pump-up sprayer should be rented or purchased. Those with long nozzles or flexible tubes are most convenient for spraying under furniture and along baseboards. The ingredients in the spray will dictate the frequency of application.

Powders or dusts have very limited use in indoor treatment. The only indications for their use is on heavily infested carpets that cannot be steam cleaned or in a dirt-covered subcellar. The entire carpet or subcellar should be covered, and the powder should be left undisturbed for as long as possible. The powder should be rubbed into the carpet fibers for longer residual effectivity; reapplications are warranted after each vacuuming.

When clients are told that their houses must be exterminated, one immediate concern is the expense of the procedure. Options include professional extermination or self-treatment of the house. If the client has a large house and if time is a priority, professional extermination is the most cost-effective, since most exterminators include retreatments in the original cost. Before the client has the house treated, the list of products to be used should be reviewed for adequacy and compatibility with the agents being used on the animals. If self-treatment is desired, a complete outline of products to use and procedures to follow should be given to the client.

OUTDOOR FLEA CONTROL

A heavily infested external environment is a source of fleas to infest the animal and, subsequently, the house. Insecticidal treatment is practical only if a small area is to be treated, but careful landscaping coupled with restrictive fencing can minimize the animal's exposure.

The grass on the property should be kept short, and the clippings and all other organic debris should be removed. The animal should be prevented from going into flower gardens, areas with tall weeds or shrubs, and shady areas. Crawl spaces under porches, houses, and kennels should be blocked off. If the animal cannot be restricted from these areas, they should be treated with an appropriate insecticide.

Yard and kennel sprays should be used for external treatment as they have been formulated for maximum residual effectiveness in all weather conditions. However, such sprays usually contain potent, toxic insecticides, so the manufacturer's instructions should be followed carefully. Additionally, all of the insecticides used to treat the animal and the house should be reviewed carefully so that the animal is not poisoned. Since yard and kennel sprays typically contain organophosphates or carbamates, botanic products should be used on the animal.

10 Miscellaneous Allergic Disorders

EAR MITE HYPERSENSITIVITY

Otoacariasis caused by *Otodectes cynotis* is common in the dog and cat. Otic symptomatology varies, ranging from none (asymptomatic) to an intense pruritus with or without exudation. Some animals will also traumatize other areas of their bodies.

Otodectes cynotis is a nonburrowing psoroptid mite that feeds on host lymph and whole blood. As the mite feeds, the host is exposed to mite antigens and can mount an immune response to these allergens. Powell demonstrated the presence of IgE-like reagin in cats experimentally infected with *Otodectes cynotis*. These cats showed immediate but not delayed skin test reactions when tested with mite extracts. After 35 days of exposure, two-hour skin test reactions occurred, which had histologic features of an Arthus (type III) reaction. Serum-precipitating antibodies were noted by day 45.

These data show that cats and probably dogs can become hypersensitive to the ear mite. Asymptomatic animals probably are not allergic, while severely pruritic animals are hypersensitive.

SARCOPTES SCABIEI HYPERSENSITIVITY

Humans infected with scabies mites remain symptom-free for approximately four weeks before developing lesions and pruritus. Symptoms can persist for one to two weeks after the mites are eradicated. When these treated patients are reinfected, only 40 percent develop clinical disease and the signs can occur within 24 hours of exposure. These clinical data suggest that an allergic sensitization plays a role in this disorder and that the allergy may be protective.

Humans will show an immediate skin test reaction to scabies extract if they have had the disease within one year of testing. Delayed hypersensitivity skin test reactions can also be seen. These results, coupled with the demonstration of circulating immune complexes and altered immunoglobulin levels, support an allergic component in this disease.

Scabies mites are burrowing acarids that are exposed to the host's immune system. Dogs with sarcoptic mange typically scratch well out of proportion to the number of mites present, have a significant peripheral lymphadenopathy, and respond poorly to steroid therapy. Asymptomatic carriers can also be identified. These findings combined with the demonstration of an eosinophilia, proteinuria, or immune complex glomerulonephritis in some dogs strongly support the theory that dogs can also become hypersensitive to the scabies mite.

INTERNAL PARASITE HYPERSENSITIVITY

IgE is thought of as an antiparasitic and antiallergenic antibody, and its production in response to ascarids and other parasites is a well-known phenomenon. Halliwell demonstrated that antiascarid IgE molecules bind to skin and other mast cells. Hirshman and others have noted an airway hypersensitivity to ascarid antigen in dogs. Butler reported that dogs naturally or experimentally sensitized to ascarid antigen developed both respiratory and cutaneous allergic reactions when challenged with antigen. Accordingly, parasitized animals may show signs of cutaneous allergy. Parasites without a larval migratory phase (whipworms and tapeworms) would not be as allergenic as parasites that migrate through the tissues (roundworms, hookworms, and heartworms).

Allergic reactions to internal parasites can vary from urticaria to a generalized lesional or nonlesional pruritus. Dogs sensitized to hookworms can develop generalized disease or focal lesions at the site of larval penetration. Heartworm infection has been associated with a pruritic nodular disease of the head, trunk, and limbs, atopic-like pruritus, and scabies-like pruritus.

In internal parasite hypersensitivity, the patient is shown to be infected by an appropriate test, and the signs resolve spontaneously when the parasite is eliminated. This supports but does not prove the allergic basis of the disorder. Since antigens to these various parasites are not available commercially, clinical documentation is impossible. All allergic patients should be checked for internal parasites, and if they are present, the animal should be treated for them before the allergy workup progresses.

OTHER PARASITE HYPERSENSITIVITIES

Virtually any insect can cause an allergic response in an individual. In humans, the caddis fly and mayfly can cause allergic reactions without direct contact. These flies lose parts of their exoskeletons, which then act as aeroallergens for some individuals in the area. Vollset reported a high incidence of allergic sensitization in dogs fed a food contaminated by storage mites. Allergic reactions to tick bites also have been reported in the dog. If it is known that the animal has been exposed to an insect, insect hypersensitivity should be suspected. Unfortunately, animals can be unknowingly exposed to parasites, for example, food storage mites, and their allergic disease can defy detection.

HORMONAL HYPERSENSITIVITY

Hormonal hypersensitivity is a rare, presumably allergic condition in which an animal becomes hypersensitive to its own endogenous sex hormones. It occurs in both males and females, but because of the cyclic variation in sex hormone levels in the bitch, it is most commonly recognized in female dogs.

As in other allergic conditions, pruritus is the clinical sign of this disorder. Initially, there is nonlesional pruritus of the lower back, perineum, and posteromedial thighs (Figs. 10–1 and 10–2). As the itching usually is fairly intense, secondary changes are common. In females, the signs start around a heat period or an overt pseudocyesis and stop when this reproductive event is over. Typical of allergic disorders, the next exposure produces more intense signs that last longer. Some bitches will become so sensitive that the signs will be continuous although estral exacerbations are recognized. Males show nonseasonal signs that intensify with time. Chronically affected animals will traumatize their faces, feet, and axillary regions as well as the posterior parts of their bodies.

Early on, the condition in these animals is easily confused with that in dogs that are food or flea hypersensitive. As the signs progress, atopic disease must also be considered. Helpful diagnostic clues for hormonal hypersensitivity include the onset or worsening of clinical signs at the time of a reproductive event and a variable resistance to glucocorticoid therapy. As was discussed before, chronically allergic dogs do not respond to steroid therapy as well as newly allergic dogs, and the response to steroids varies in food hypersensitivity. Animals with a hormonal hypersensitivity tend to respond poorly to adequate steroid therapy; this is unusual in an early inhalant- or flea-allergic animal.

The definitive documentation of a hormonal hypersensitivity is currently impossible. In the past, skin testing with aqueous solutions of estrogen, progesterone, and testosterone was advocated, but these hormones are expensive and difficult to obtain, so testing is not routinely done. The diagnosis is supported by the elimination of all the appropriate differential diagnoses and by the animal's response

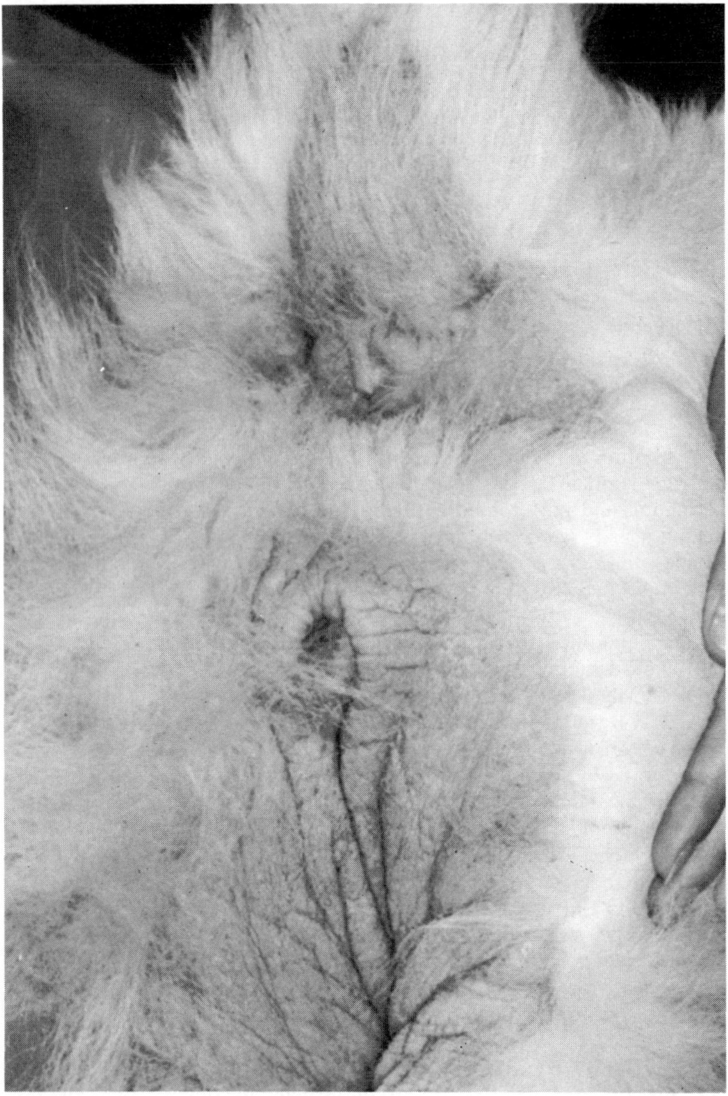

FIGURE 10–1. Alopecia, erythema, and lichenification of the perineal skin.

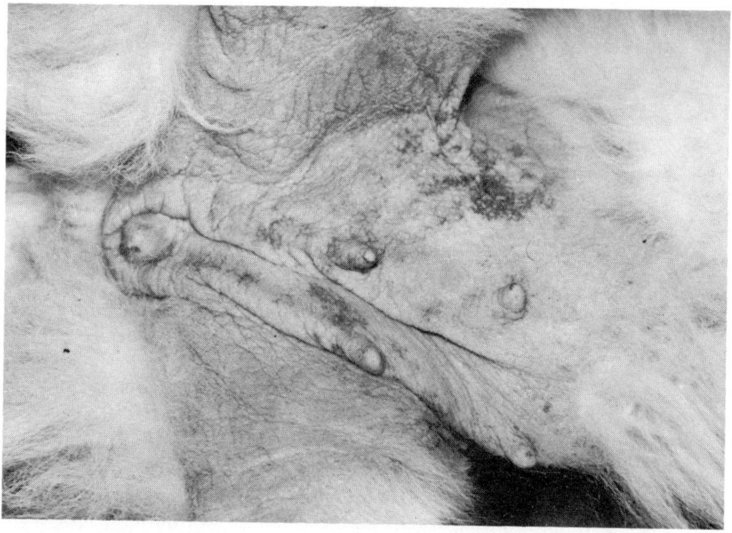

FIGURE 10–2. Alopecia, erythema, and lichenification of the ventral abdomen, medial thighs, and vulvar area.

to neutering. After surgery, most dogs show significant improvement within two weeks. If a female dog is a breeding bitch or if the owners are reluctant to neuter the dog without an absolute diagnosis, oral or repositol testosterone should be administered at a dose of 0.5 to 1.0 mg/kg to a maximum level of 30 mg. The bitch with hormonal hypersensitivity should stop scratching with this drug, and the signs should recur when the drug is withdrawn. The testosterone administration should be used as a presurgical diagnostic test and not for long-term management. In males, the testosterone test is unproven. As testosterone is likely to be the offending hormone, administration of this drug should aggravate the condition, while progestational therapy should decrease the pruritus. Therapy consists of neutering the animal.

BACTERIAL HYPERSENSITIVITY

Bacterial infections of the skin are common in the dog, and there is usually some underlying dermatologic disorder that predisposes the dog to infection. Most dogs with pyodermas are pruritic to some degree, and the pruritus should stop with appropriate antibiotic therapy. Pathologic pruritus is triggered by a variety of mediators that include histamine, proteolytic enzymes, kallikrein, and bradykinin. In staphylococcal skin infections, antibody production for opsonization and neutrophil phagocytosis and killing is important for the elimination of the organisms. Proteolytic enzymes released from the neutrophils or other modulators generated through the humoral amplification system cause the infected skin to itch. When dogs with superficial pyodermas are treated with glucocorticoids, their pruritus usually disappears, while the rash improves but does not completely resolve. The improvement seen is due to the decrease in inflammation. When the drug is discontinued, the pyoderma and pruritus will recur and will be more severe and more difficult to treat.

Although Walton first introduced the concept of clinical bacterial allergy in dogs in 1966, Baker was the first investigator to describe staphylococcal allergy. Baker stated that dogs with a bacterial allergy could present with an obvious pyoderma or as classically allergic with or without an obvious infection. The dogs with the allergic presentation showed secondary eczematoid and seborrheic changes and hair loss. Some dogs also had blepharitis and iritis. The history from these animals often indicated that the dog had a previous staphylococcal infection that presumably sensitized the dog. Baker proposed that unapparent staphylococcal infections of the tonsils, anal sacs, or internal organs acted as sources of antigen release in dogs with no obvious skin infection. Colonization of normal skin must also be considered.

The work of Baker, Breen, and Scott has led to the description of the clinical lesions associated with staphylococcal hypersensitivity—the erythematous pustule, the hemorrhagic vesicle or bulla, and the patch of seborrheic dermatitis. The erythematous pustule is a follicular papule or pustule with a large erythematous halo. The hemorrhagic bulla, shown in Figure 10–3, also has a ring of peripheral erythema. The seborrheic patch varies in appearance. Small lesions are annular areas of hair loss and erythema that expand peripherally with inflammation and peeling (epidermal collarette) at the leading edge (Fig. 10–4). As the lesion ages, its size increases and the central erythema fades and often becomes hyperpigmented. Lesions can coalesce and form large areas of hair loss that centrally look inactive (Fig. 10–5). Examination of the leading edge of the hair loss will indicate active inflammation. Rarely, one will see a nonlesionally pruritic allergic dog that is allergic to staphylococcal antigens from unapparent infections, especially of the anal sacs.

None of the lesions associated with staphylococcal hypersensitivity are pathognomonic for this condition. The erythematous pustule and seborrheic patch are often seen in dogs with pyodermas in which there is no evidence of a staphylococcal hypersensitivity. The hemorrhagic bulla is much more suggestive of staphylococcal hypersensitivity but also can be seen in dogs with a vasculitis. The animal's history helps support the tentative diagnosis of a bacterial allergy. The animal's pruritus is not lessened with appropriate glucocorticoid therapy but stops with prolonged antibiotic therapy. As was dis-

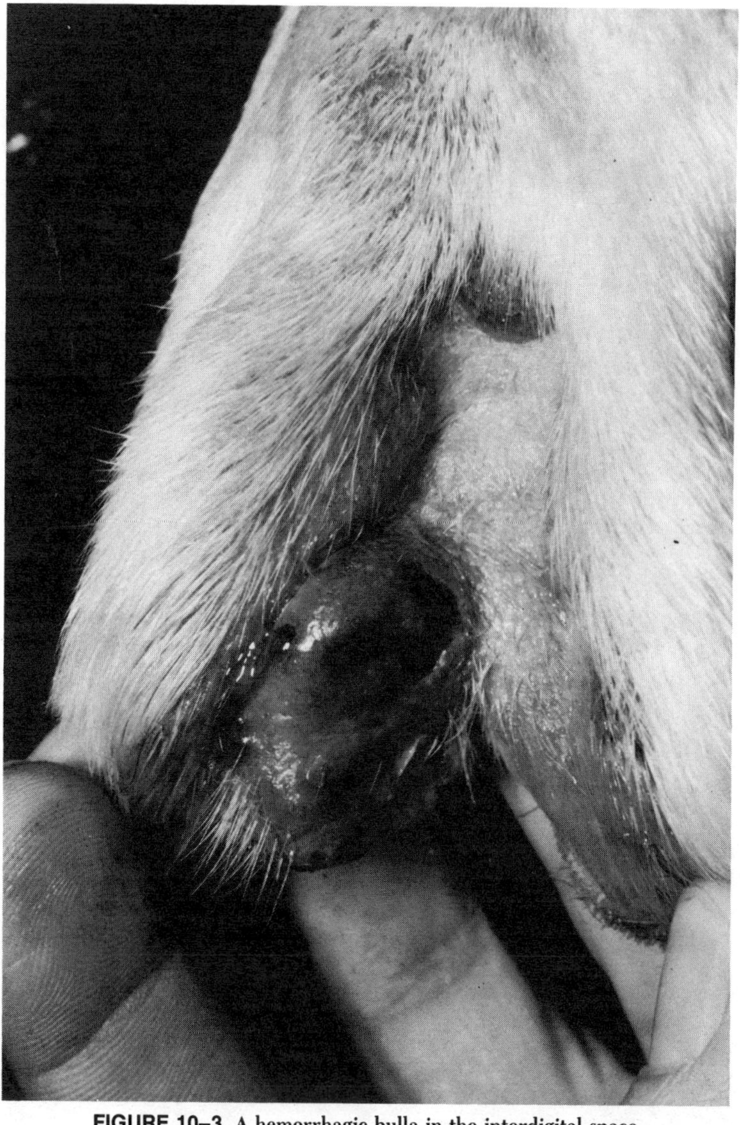

FIGURE 10–3. A hemorrhagic bulla in the interdigital space.

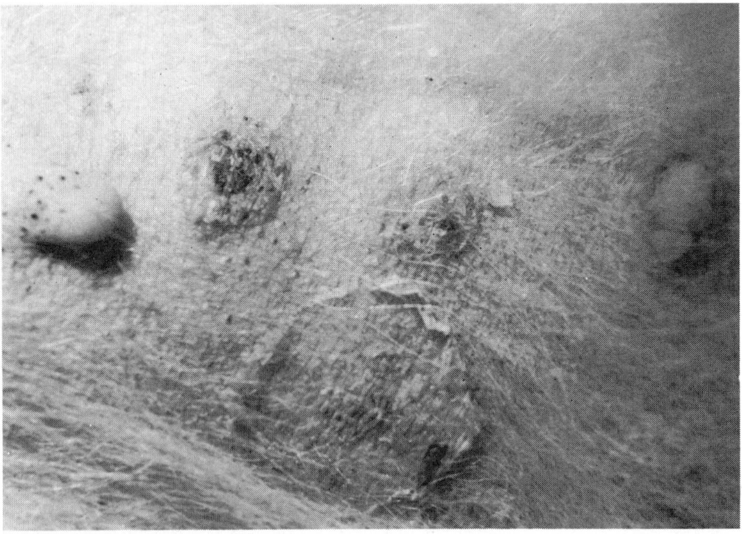

FIGURE 10–4. Focal areas of bacterial hypersensitivity with epidermal collarettes.

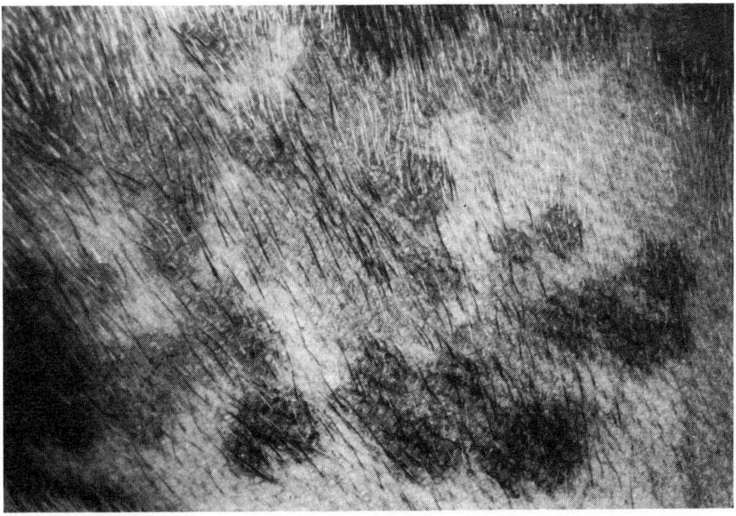

FIGURE 10–5. Coalescence of individual lesions into a larger area.

cussed before, routine infections can also be pruritic, so response to antibacterial therapy is not diagnostic. The dog with a staphylococcal hypersensitivity should remain normal for some period of time after the antibiotics are discontinued but can spontaneously develop new lesions in normal skin or start to scratch at normal skin. Signs typically recur within 30 to 60 days. Dogs that develop new lesions in areas of diseased skin may have a staphylococcal hypersensitivity superimposed on some other condition or may simply be experiencing a recurrent pyoderma secondary to some other problem. Nonlesionally pruritic dogs that stop scratching when given antibiotic therapy and that return to scratching when the drug is discontinued are strong candidates for the diagnosis of a bacterial allergy.

The history and physical findings can strongly support the tentative diagnosis of staphylococcal hypersensitivity, but the confirmation of the diagnosis requires skin biopsies or skin testing or both. The biopsy results vary with the nature of the clinical lesion, and the vascular changes are of critical importance. The erythematous pustule and hemorrhagic bulla show signs of vascular inflammation with extravasation of red blood cells or dermal hemorrhage. These findings are not typical of nonallergic pyodermas. The seborrheic lesions tend to show more vascular dilatation and neutrophilic infiltration but can be indistinguishable from other seborrheic lesions.

Skin testing typically has been done with a staphylococcal cell wall antigen and toxoid mixture (Staphoid A-B, manufactured by Coopers Animal Health, Kansas City, MO). One-tenth ml of the full-strength antigen or of a 50-percent dilution with saline is given intradermally and the test is read immediately (15 to 30 minutes) and at 24 and 48 hours. All dogs will show immediate reactions characterized by erythematous wheals varying from 14 to 20 mm in diameter. In nonallergic dogs, the lesions fade slowly and an indurated, occasionally erythematous nodule of 5 to 9 mm in diameter will remain at the late readings. In hypersensitive dogs, the delayed reactions are very inflammatory and vary in size from 9 to 75 mm. The lesions are not wheals but rather are erythematous, indurated, oozing nodules that may become necrotic (Fig. 10–6). Biopsies of these lesions typically show signs of a vasculitis.

The diagnosis of staphylococcal hypersensitivity does not necessarily mean that the dog will need specific therapy. Diseased skin is easily infected, and recurrent infections can sensitize the animal. If the dog has some underlying disease that can be identified and treated, resolution of the primary disorder coupled with prolonged (four to eight week) antibiotic therapy may "cure" the dog. Scott reported that 45 percent of his 31 cases fell into this category. The hypersensitivity in these animals would persist for some time, but the normalization of the skin would eliminate or minimize the animal's exposure to the antigen.

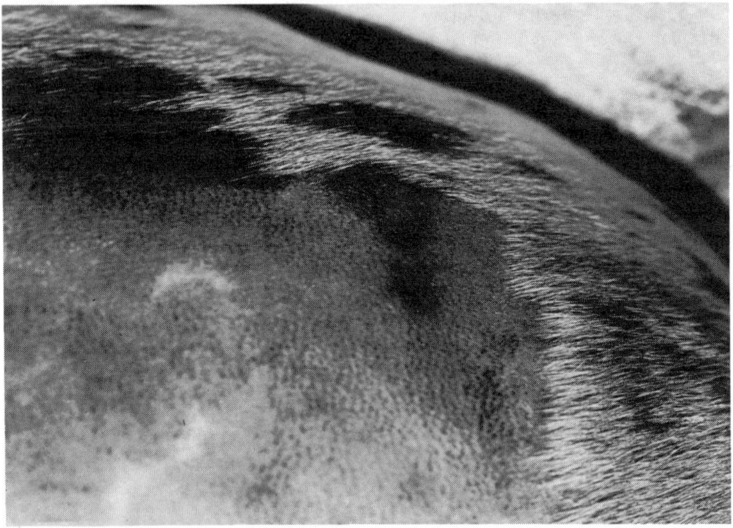

FIGURE 10–6. A focal area of necrosis at the site of a Staphoid A-B skin test—36-hour reading.

Dogs that have a staphylococcal hypersensitivity for no apparent reason or that do not "self-cure" with the resolution of the underlying disease will require long-term, presumably lifelong therapy. Therapy can consist of antibiotics or staphylococcal vaccines. The ideal method of treatment is immunotherapy. Animals that do not respond to the immunotherapy may be controlled with long-term antibiotic therapy.

Long-term antibiotic therapy can involve the periodic use of full-dose therapy or the constant use of a low dose of the drug. If the animal's episodes of disease are separated by long intervals of normalcy, each episode should be treated until the infection is completely resolved, and then the drug should be discontinued. This pattern is unusual. Animals typically remain normal for only relatively short periods; thus the need for antibiotic therapy is almost constant. In this situation, the dog should be treated on a maintenance basis with one daily dose of a drug or with the full therapeutic dose once or twice weekly. For example, a 50-pound dog could be treated with cephalexin (Keflex) at a dose of 500 mg once daily or 500 mg twice daily one or two days of the week. Chronic antibiotic therapy can be expensive and could lead to bacterial resistance, chronic intoxication, altered bowel function, and drug reactions, but there may be no alternatives.

Immunotherapy is the ideal form of treatment as it appears to be safe and is relatively inexpensive. Presently, autogenous staphylococcal vaccines, staphylococcal phage lysates, and the cell wall and toxoid mixture used for testing are utilized therapeutically by various investigators. Since these products are immunostimulants, they are also used in the treatment of recurrent pyodermas secondary to immunodeficiencies. These bacterial antigens are probably antigenically dissimilar and are used in different ways to treat various diseases in dogs. Accordingly, it is difficult if not impossible to state an accurate success rate of therapy for staphylococcal hypersensitivity.

Baker described a protocol for use with Staphoid A-B (50% dilution), which is as follows:

DAY	TOTAL DOSE (ml)	INTRADERMAL DOSE (ml)	NONINTRADERMAL DOSE (ml)
1	0.25	0.1	0.15
2	0.50	0.1	0.40
3	0.75	0.1	0.65
4	1.00	0.1	0.90
5	1.25	0.1	1.15
12	1.50	0.1	1.40
19	1.75	0.1	1.65
26	2.00	0.1	1.90

He gave the nonintradermal dose either subcutaneously or half intramuscularly and half subcutaneously. He reported that this therapy was uniformly effective, and that one course of therapy was usually sufficient, although some dogs need periodic booster injections.

Scott followed Baker's protocol and successfully treated six out of nine dogs. All of these dogs needed booster injections every one to three months. Pukay used a very similar protocol in which the dose at day 19 and 26 was 1.50 ml, and he noted an excellent response in 14 of his 16 cases. Forty-four percent of the dogs that responded required a booster injection within 30 days, while the remainder required an injection within two months. Thus, the reported success rate with Baker's Staphoid A-B protocol varies between 67 and 88 percent.

Other investigators use different bacterial antigens, especially Staphage Lysate, to treat dogs with recurrent pyodermas and report that success rates do not exceed 50 percent. Unfortunately, it is unclear whether these patients are staphylococcal hypersensitive or whether they develop recurrent pyodermas for other reasons.

Investigators who use Staphage Lysate or autogenous bacterins typically give weekly subcutaneous injections with gradually increasing doses of 0.1 or 0.25 ml until the maintenance dose of either 0.5 or 1.0 ml is reached. For large dogs, one author (WHM) gives incremental doses of 0.2 ml every other day until the final dose of

1.0 ml is reached and has not seen any adverse reactions to this accelerated schedule. Maintenance injections are given once weekly. Animals that do not respond after two months of maintenance therapy are not likely to do so. Dogs that respond to the weekly injections may be maintained with less frequent injections.

In summary, although pyodermas are common, bacterial hypersensitivity appears to be rare. Resolution of any underlying dermatologic condition may result in a self-cure of the bacterial allergy. Based on the available data, Staphoid A-B appears to be an effective antigen that causes very few side effects. Local Arthus-like reactions initially will be seen at the site of the intradermal injection, but the reactivity will subside with time. Some dogs will show irritant or allergic reactions to the subcutaneous dose, and in these animals, that injection is eliminated while the intradermal injection is continued.

DRUG REACTIONS

Drugs are low molecular weight compounds that can produce side effects of an expected or unexpected nature. Although expected drug reactions can be undesirable, such as the hair loss associated with the use of some chemotherapeutic agents, the reactions are attributed to the drug's pharmacologic or physiologic effect. Unexpected reactions that affect the skin are called drug eruptions, and they can have an immunologic or a nonimmunologic basis. In humans, it is estimated that drug eruptions will occur in 2 to 3 percent of hospitalized patients. Reports of drug eruptions in animals are infrequent but probably are more common than the literature would indicate.

Drug eruptions can be caused by impurities in the drug, drug metabolites, binding agents (such as starches and stearates), and flavoring agents. Molecules of increased size and complexity are more immunogenic, and drugs that contain proteins can be more allergenic. Since most drugs are haptens, they must bind to host proteins before they become allergenic. Drugs that bind easily to proteins are more likely to cause drug eruptions.

Aside from the nature of the drug, other factors that influence the frequency of drug eruptions include the dose, route of administration, previous administration of the drug, and previous drug allergies. The possibility of a drug eruption is increased by the simultaneous local and systemic administration of the same drug, intermittent use of the drug, or use of a repositol form of the drug. In humans, other risk factors include the genetic background of the patient, the nature of the disease being treated, concomitant drug therapy, and intercurrent infections. Patients with infectious mononucleosis have a 95 to 100 percent chance of developing a drug eruption if they are treated with ampicillin. These factors have not been evaluated in companion animals.

Immunologic drug eruptions do not occur at the first administration of the drug. Sensitization must first occur and usually takes at least one week. Reactions that occur in a large number of patients and that occur at the first administration are not immunologically mediated. Drug eruptions can be caused by type, I, II, III, or IV hypersensitivity reactions, and although certain drugs typically cause one type of reaction, there is no specific reaction pattern for any one drug. In humans, maculopapular rashes and urticarial reactions are the most common manifestations of a drug eruption. Less common reaction patterns include fixed drug eruptions, contact dermatitis, erythema multiforme, toxic epidermal necrolysis, pemphigus-like eruptions, lupus-like eruptions, vasculitis, and photosensitization. Except for the fixed drug eruption, these reactive patterns have a sudden onset and are symmetrical and widespread.

The list of drugs known to cause drug eruptions in humans is extensive. Drugs from these lists which are frequently used in companion animal medicine are the penicillins,* cephalosporins,* chloramphenicol,* sulfa drugs,* griseofulvin,* barbiturates,* phenytoins,* phenylbutazone, aspirin, furosemide, neomycin,* and topical anesthetics.* Less commonly used drugs include phenothiazine,* propylthiouracil,* gold salts,* female sex hormones,* dapsone,* quinidine,* thiabendazole,* and nystatin. Other drugs reported to cause reactions in dogs and cats include 5-fluorocytosine, diethylcarbamazine, thiacetarsamide, levamisole, prednisolone, thyroid extract, gentamicin, and a variety of topical products, vaccines, bacterins, and antisera.

In animals, drug allergies typically are eruptive processes that can be painful or pruritic. Noneruptive pruritus mimicking atopy or food hypersensitivity has been associated with thyroid extract, diethylcarbamazine, and flavoring agents in vitamins and heartworm preventives. Unless the drug reaction causes an urticarial reaction or a noneruptive pruritus, drug allergy is often overlooked.

The lesions of a drug eruption can mimic any known dermatosis and can be papular, exfoliative, vesiculobullous, erythrodermatous, purpuric, or ulcerative. Alopecic conditions and fixed drug eruptions occasionally will be seen. As in humans, the papular form appears to be the most common.

To diagnose a drug eruption, one must have an index of suspicion, since this reaction can mimic many skin conditions. A careful history about all medications and nutritional supplements is critical. After the initial sensitization period, drug eruptions can occur at any time during administration and may even occur a few days after the drug

*These drugs have been reported to cause eruptions in companion animals.

is discontinued. Thus, if an animal has a drug history, a drug hypersensitivity may be present. Animals that are being treated for a dermatologic condition can be difficult to evaluate. If the owner reports that the condition was initially responding to the medication but then suddenly worsened, a drug eruption may have been superimposed upon the original condition.

Presently, there are no reliable specific tests to document a drug allergy. Spontaneous resolution of the eruption with drug withdrawal implicates the drug as a causative factor but does not prove the immunologic basis. Drug challenge would further strengthen the definitive diagnosis but is not advised as the next reaction could be much more severe. Skin biopsies will help eliminate other diseases from consideration and can strongly support diagnosis of a drug eruption.

If a drug eruption is suspected, the drug should be discontinued. If the animal is receiving multiple drugs, they all should be discontinued, but if that is not possible, the last drug added would be most suspect. With drug withdrawal, drug eruptions typically resolve spontaneously in 7 to 14 days, although they can last longer. Animals with serious reactions, such as toxic epidermal necrolysis, will require intensive supportive care. In those animals in which a drug eruption has been documented, prophylaxis is of utmost importance. Readministration of that drug or a similar one could cause a much more serious reaction. Patients allergic to penicillin should not be treated with any other member of the penicillin family, and cephalosporins should be used cautiously as these drugs contain the β-lactam ring found in penicillin.

Bibliography

CHAPTER 1

Fitzpatrick, T.B., Eisen, A.Z., Wolff, K., et al (eds): Dermatology in General Medicine (ed 3). New York, McGraw-Hill, 1987, pp 400–410, 426–442.

Fundenberg, H.H., Stites, D.P., Caldwell, J.L., and Wells, J.V. (eds): Basic and Clinical Immunology (ed 3). Los Altos, Lange Medical Publications, 1980, pp 1–8, 16–43, 64–78.

Gell, P.G.H., Coombs, R.R.A., and Lockman, P.J.: Clinical Aspects of Immunology (ed 3). Oxford, Blackwell Scientific Publications, 1977.

Halliwell, R.E.W.: The immunology of allergic skin disease. J Small Anim Pract 12:431–443, 1971.

Halliwell, R.E.W.: The localization of IgE in canine skin: An immunofluorescent study. J Immunol 110:422–430, 1973.

Halliwell, R.E.W., Fleischman, J.B., et al: The role of allergy in chronic pulmonary disease in horses. J Am Vet Med Assoc 174:277–281, 1979.

Humphrey, J.H., and White, R.G.: Immunology for Students of Medicine (ed 2). Los Altos, Lange Medical Publications, 1978.

Middleton, E., Reed, C.E., and Ellis, E.F. (eds): Allergy: Principles and Practices (ed 2). St. Louis, C.V. Mosby Company, 1983.

Muller, G.H., Kirk, R.W., and Scott, D.W.: Small Animal Dermatology (ed 3). Philadelphia, W.B. Saunders Company, 1983, pp 380–400.

Richet C.: Anaphylaxis. Translated by J.M. Bligh. Constable, London, Liverpool University Press, 1913.

Rola-Pleszczynski, M.: Immunoregulation by leukotrienes and other lipoxygenase metabolites. Immunol Today 6:303–307, 1985.

Stone, J. (ed): Dermatologic Immunology and Allergy. St. Louis, C.V. Mosby Company, 1985, pp 3–13, 27–37, 53–123, 179–209.

Tizard, I.: An Introduction to Veterinary Immunology (ed 2). Philadelphia, W.B. Saunders Company, 1982.

Tizard, I.: Basic immunology. 2: Reviewing the properties of antibodies. Vet Med 81:166–178, 1986.

Voorhees, J.J.: Leukotrienes and other lipoxygenase products in the pathogenesis and therapy of psoriasis and other dermatoses. Arch Dermatol 119:541–547, 1983.

Wittich, F.W.: Spontaneous allergy (atopy) in the lower animal: Seasonal hay fever (fall type) in a dog. J Allergy 12:247–251, 1941.

CHAPTER 2

Butler, J.M., Peters, J.E., et al: Pruritic dermatitis in asthmatic Basenji-Greyhound dogs: A model for human atopic dermatitis. J Am Acad Dermatol 8:33–38, 1983.

Frick, O.L.: Immediate hypersensitivity. *In* Fundenberg, H.H., Stites, D.P., Caldwell, J.L., and Wells, J.V. (eds): Basic and Clinical Immunology (ed 3). Los Altos, Lange Medical Publications, 1980, pp 274–295.

Frick, O.L., and Brooks, D.L.: Immunoglobulin E antibodies to pollens augmented in dogs by virus vaccines. Am J Vet Res 44:440–445, 1983.

Greenberger, P.A.: Classification of hypersensitivity reactions, Arthus reactions and beta-blockade theory. *In* Stone, J. (ed): Dermatologic Immunology and Allergy. St. Louis, C.V. Mosby Company, 1985, pp 287–296.

Gross, T.E., Kwochka, K.W., and Kunkle, G.A.: Correlation of histologic and immunologic findings in cats with miliary dermatitis. J Am Vet Med Assoc 189:1322–1325, 1986.

Halliwell, R.E.W.: The localization of IgE in canine skin: An immunofluorescent study. J Immunol 110:422–430, 1973.

Halliwell, R.E.W.: The sites of production and localization of IgE in canine tissues. Ann NY Acad Sci 254:476–488, 1975.

Halliwell, R.E.W.: Hyposensitization in the treatment of atopic disease. *In* Kirk, R.W. (ed): Current Veterinary Therapy VI. Philadelphia, W.B. Saunders Company, 1977, pp 537–541.

Hirshman, C.A., Downes, H., et al: Basenji-Greyhound dog model of asthma: Pulmonary responses after beta-adrenergic blockade. J Appl Physiol 51:1423–1427, 1981.

Katz, D.H.: The immune system: An overview. *In* Fundenberg, H.H., Stites, D.P., Caldwell, J.L., and Wells, J.V. (eds): Basic and Clinical Immunology (ed 3). Los Altos, Lange Medical Publications, 1980, pp 1–8.

Marsh, D.G., Bias, W.B., and Ishizaka, K.: Genetic control of basal serum immunoglobulin E level and its effect on specific reaginic sensitivity. Proc Natl Acad Sci USA 71:3588–3592, 1974.

Muller, G.H., Kirk, R.W., and Scott, D.W.: Small Animal Dermatology (ed 3). Philadelphia, W.B. Saunders Company, 1983, pp 400–415.

Nesbitt, G.H., Kedan, G.S., and Caciolo, P.: Canine atopy. Part I: Etiology and diagnosis. Comp Cont Ed 6:73–84, 1984.

Phillips, T.M.: Biochemistry of the immune system. *In* Stone, J. (ed): Dermatologic Immunology and Allergy. St. Louis, C.V. Mosby Company, 1985, pp 81–101.

Reedy, L.M.: Canine atopy. Comp Cont Ed 1:550–556, 1979.

Schick, R.O., and Fadok, V.A.: Response of atopic dogs to regional allergens: 268 cases (1981–1984). J Am Vet Med Asoc 189:1493–1496, 1986.

Schwartzman, R.M., Massicot, J.G., et al: The atopic dog model: Report of an attempt to establish a colony. Int Arch Allergy Appl Immunol 72:97–101, 1983.

Schwartzman, R.M.: Immunologic studies of progeny of atopic dogs. Am J Vet Res 45:375–378, 1984.

Scott, D.W.: Observations on canine atopy. J Am Anim Hosp Assoc 17:91–100, 1981.

Scott, D.W., Walton, D.K., and Slater, M.R.: Miliary dermatitis. A feline cutaneous reaction pattern. Proceedings of the Second Annual Kal Kan Seminar, Eastern States Veterinary Conference, Orlando, 1986, pp 11–18.

Sherman, B.V., and Monroe, E.W.: Urticaria and angioedema. *In* Stone, J. (ed): Dermatologic Immunology and Allergy. St. Louis, C.V. Mosby Company, 1985, pp 333–351.

Szentivanyi, A.: Beta-adrenergic theory of the atopic abnormality in bronchial asthma. J Allergy Clin Immunol 42:203–232, 1968.

Terr, A.I.: Allergic diseases. *In* Fundenberg, H.H., Stites, D.P., Caldwell, J.L., and Wells, J.V. (eds): Basic and Clinical Immunology (ed 3). Los Altos, Lange Medical Publications, 1980, pp 513–531.

Van Stee, E.W.: Risk factors in canine atopy. Calif Vet 4:8–10, 1983.

Vollset, I.: Atopic dermatitis in Norwegian dogs. Nord Vet Med 37:97–106, 1985.

Vriesendorp, H.M., Smid-Merex, B.M.J., et al: Serological DL-A typing of normal and atopic dogs. Transplant Proc 7:375–377, 1975.

Wasserman, S.I.: The mast cell and its mediators. *In* Stone, J. (ed): Dermatologic Immunology and Allergy. St. Louis, C.V. Mosby Company, 1985, pp 187–196.

Wells, J.V.: Immune mechanisms in tissue damage. *In* Fundenberg, H.H., Stites, D.P., Caldwell, J.L., and Wells, J.V. (eds): Basic and Clinical Immunology (ed 3). Los Altos, Lange Medical Publications, 1980, pp 191–206.

Willemse, A., and Van den Brom, W.E.: Evaluation of the intradermal allergy test in normal dogs. Res Vet Sci 32:57–61, 1982.

Willemse, A., and Van den Brom, W.E.: Investigations of the symptomatology and significance of immediate skin test reactivity in canine atopic dermatitis. Res Vet Sci 34:261–265, 1983.

Willemse, A., Noordzij, A., et al: Allergen specific IgG_d antibodies in dogs with atopic dermatitis as determined by the enzyme linked immunosorbent assay (ELISA). Clin Expl Immunol 59:359–363, 1985.

Wright, S.: Atopic dermatitis and essential fatty acids: A biochemical basis for atopy? Acta Dermatol Venerol 114:143–145, 1985.

CHAPTER 3

Anderson, M.C., and Baer, H.: Antigenic and allergenic changes during storage of pollen extract. J Allergy Clin Immunol 69:3–10, 1982.

Baer, H.: Allergenic extracts. *In* Middleton, E., Reed, C.E., and Ellis, E.F. (eds): Allergy: Principles and Practice (ed 2). St. Louis, C.V. Mosby Company, 1983, pp 255–270.

Conant, N.F., Smith, D.T., Baker, R.D., and Callaway, J.L.: Manual of Clinical Mycology (ed 3). Philadelphia, W.B. Saunders Company, 1971.

Meriney, D.K., Wallace, D., et al: Clinical comparison of skin testing and the radioallergosorbent test in dog-sensitive patients using mixed and breed-specific antigen. Int Arch Allergy Appl Immunol 58:453–459, 1979.

Nelson, H.S.: Effect of preservatives and conditions of storage on the potency of allergy extracts. J Allergy Clin Immunol 67:64–69, 1981.

Nesbitt, G.H.: Canine allergic inhalant dermatitis: A review of 230 cases. J Am Vet Med Assoc 172:55–60, 1978.

Nesbitt, G.H., Caciolo, P., and Kedan, G.S.: Aeroallergens. Comp Cont Ed 6:63–68, 1984.

Nesbitt, G.H., Kedan, G.S., and Caciolo, P.: Canine atopy. Part I: Etiology and diagnosis. Comp Cont Ed 6:73–84, 1984.

Nesbitt, G.H., Kedan, G.S., and Caciolo, P.: Canine atopy. Part II: Management. Comp Cont Ed 6:264–275, 1984.

Ohman, J.L., Baer, H., Anderson, M.C., et al: Surface washes of living cats: An improved method of obtaining clinically relevant allergen. J Allergy Clin Immunol 72:288–293, 1983.

Schick, R.O., and Fadok, V.A.: Response of atopic dogs to regional allergens: 268 cases (1981–1984). J Am Vet Med Assoc 189:1493–1496, 1986.

Scott, D.W.: Observations on canine atopy. J Am Anim Hosp Assoc 17:91–100, 1981.

Solomon, W.R., and Mathews, K.P.: Aerobiology and inhalant allergens. *In* Middleton, E., Reed, C.E., and Ellis, E.F. (eds): Allergy: Principles and Practice (ed 2). St. Louis, C. V. Mosby Company, 1973, pp 1143–1202.

Terracina, F., and Rogers, S.A.: In-home fungal studies: Methods to increase the yield. Ann Allergy 49:35–37, 1982.

Tufts, L.: Allergy Management in Clinical Practice. St. Louis, C.V. Mosby Company, 1973.

Vollset, I.: Immediate type hypersensitivity in dogs induced by storage mites. Res Vet Sci 40:123–127, 1986.

Weber, R.W.: Cross-reactivity among pollens. Ann Allergy 46:208–215, 1981.

CHAPTER 4

August, J.R.: The reaction of canine skin to the intradermal injection of allergic extracts. J Am Anim Hosp Assoc 18:157–171, 1982.

Barbet, J.: Hydroxyzine withdrawal time for intradermal testing in dogs. Proceedings of the Annual AAVD and ACVD, 1987, p 21.

Bioproducts DVM, Inc.: A micro-ELISA assay for measurement of allergen-specific IgE antibodies in canines, 1987.

Dockhorn, R.J., Grater, W.C., and Mitchell, W.R.: Report from the committee on standardization of the American College of Allergists. Ann Allergy 38:129–133, 1977.

Halliwell, R.E.W., and Kunkle, G.A.: The radioallergosorbent test in the diagnosis of canine atopic disease. J Allergy Clin Immunol 62:236–242, 1978.

Johansson, S.G.O., and Foucard, T.: IgE in immunity and disease. *In* Middleton, E., Reed, C.E., and Ellis, E.F. (eds): Allergy: Principles and Practice. St. Louis, C.V. Mosby Company, 1978, pp 551–562.

Muller, G.H., Kirk, R.W., and Scott, D.W.: Small Animal Dermatology (ed 3). Philadelphia, W.B. Saunders Company, 1983, pp 402–415.

Nelson H.S.: Diagnostic procedures in allergy: Allergy skin testing. Ann Allergy 51:411–417, 1983.

Nesbitt, G.H., Kedan, G.S., and Caciolo, P.: Canine atopy. Part I: Etiology and diagnosis. Comp Cont Ed 6:75–84, 1984.

Schwartzman, R.M.: Immunologic studies of progeny of atopic dogs. Am J Vet Res 45:375–378, 1984.

Scott, D.W.: Observations on canine atopy. J Am Anim Hosp Assoc 17:91–100, 1981.

Shirk, M.E.: The canine RAST: A diagnostic procedure for allergy inhalant dermatitis. Proceedings of the Annual AAVD and ACVD, 1986, p 32.

Van Stee, E.W.: Compound 48/80 in routine skin testing for canine allergy. Vet Med Small Anim Clin 77:1081–1086, 1982.

Vollset, I.: Atopic dermatitis in Norwegian dogs. Nord Vet Med 37:97–106, 1985.

Willemse, A., and Van den Brom, W.E.: Evaluation of the intradermal allergy test in normal dogs. Res Vet Sci 32:57–61, 1982.

Willemse, A., and Van den Brom, W.E.: Investigations of the symptomatology and the significance of immediate skin test reactivity in canine atopic dermatitis. Res Vet Sci 34:261–265, 1983.

Willemse, A., Noordzij, A., Van den Brom, W.E., and Rutten, V.P.M.G.: Allergen specific IgG_d antibodies in dogs with atopic dermatitis as determined by the enzyme linked immunosorbent assay (ELISA). Clin Expl Immunol 59:359–363, 1985.

CHAPTER 5

Anderson, W.: Canine Allergic Inhalant Dermatitis. St. Louis, Ralston Purina Company, 1975.

Baker, E.: Management of allergic disease by hyposensitization. J Am Vet Med Assoc 154:491–494, 1969.

Chamberlain, K.W.: Biological management of the allergic patient. Vet Clin North Am 4:65–77, 1978.

Greenberger, P.A.: Asthma and allergic rhinitis. *In* Stone, J. (ed): Dermatologic Immunology and Allergy. St. Louis, C.V. Mosby Company, 1985, pp 323–332.

Halliwell, R.E.W.: Hyposensitization in the treatment of atopic disease. *In* Kirk, R.W. (ed): Current Veterinary Therapy VI. Philadelphia, W.B. Saunders Company, 1977, pp 537–541.

Halliwell, R.E.W.: Hyposensitization in the treatment of flea bite hypersensitivity: Results of a double-blinded study. J Am Anim Hosp Assoc 17:249–253, 1981.

Ishizaka, K.: Possible approaches to turn off the IgE response. Ann Allergy 47:162–165, 1981.

Kunkle, G.A.: The treatment of canine atopic disease. *In* Kirk, R.W. (ed): Current Veterinary Therapy VII. Philadelphia, W.B. Saunders Company, 1980, pp 453–458.

Kwong, F.K.: Allergen extracts and purified allergen in immunotherapy. Ann Allergy 47:162–165, 1981.

McDougal, B.J.: Allergy testing and hyposensitization for three common feline dermatoses. Mod Vet Pract 81:629–633, 1986.

Muller, G.H., Kirk, R.W., and Scott, D.W.: Small Animal Dermatology (ed 3). Philadelphia, W.B. Saunders Company, 1983, pp 402–415.

Nagaya, H.: Long-term effects of conventional immunotherapy in southern California. Ann Allergy 44:193–199, 1980.

Neiburger, R.G., Neiburger, J.B., and Dockhorn, M.D.: Distribution of peripheral blood T and B lymphocyte markers in atopic children and changes during immunotherapy. J Allergy Clin Immunol 61:88–92, 1978.

Nelson, H.S.: Long-term immunotherapy with aqueous and alum-precipitated grass extracts. Ann Allergy 45:333–337, 1980.

Nesbitt, G.H.: Canine allergic inhalant dermatitis: A review of 230 cases. J Am Vet Med Assoc 172:55–60, 1978.

Nesbitt, G.H., Kedan, G.S., and Caciolo, P.: Canine atopy. Part II: Management. Comp Cont Ed 6:264–274, 1984.

Norman, P.S., and Lichtenstein, L.M.: The clinical and immunologic specificity of immunotherapy. J Allergy Clin Immunol 61:370–377, 1978.

Patterson, R., Lieberman, P., et al: Immunotherapy. *In* Middleton, E., Reed, C.E., and Ellis, E.F. (eds): Allergy: Principles and Practice (ed 2). St. Louis, C.V. Mosby Company, 1983, pp 1119–1142.

Reedy, L.M.: Canine atopy. Comp Cont Ed 1:550–556, 1979.

Reedy, L.M.: Results of allergy testing and hyposensitization in selected feline skin diseases. J Am Anim Hosp Assoc 18:618–623, 1982.

Roeklin, R.E., Sheffer, A.L., et al: Generation of antigen-specific suppressor cells during allergy desensitization. N Engl J Med 302:1213–1219, 1980.

Rose, B.: Immunotherapy: Areas of doubt. Med Clin North Am 58:127–133, 1974.

Scott, D.W.: Observations on canine atopy. J Am Anim Hosp Assoc 17:91–100, 1981.

Scott, D.W., Walton, D.K., and Slater, M.R.: Miliary dermatitis: A feline cutaneous reaction pattern. Proceedings of the 2nd Annual Kal Kan Seminar, Eastern States Veterinary Conference, Orlando, 1986, pp 11–18.

Shirk, M.E.: The canine RAST: A diagnostic procedure for allergy inhalant dermatitis. Proceedings of the Annual AAVD and ACVD, 1986, p 32.

Tipton, W.R.: Experience with daily immunotherapy in 59 adult allergic patients. J Allergy Clin Immunol 69:194–199, 1982.

Willemse, A., Van den Brom, W.E., and Rijnberk, A.: Effect of hyposensitization on atopic dermatitis in dogs. J Am Vet Med Assoc 184:1277–1280, 1984.

Wladbott, G.L.: Immunotherapy, can we improve it? Ann Allergy 45:56–58, 1980.

CHAPTER 6

Jenkins, W.L.: Pharmacologic control of inflammation. *In* Davis, L.E. (ed): Handbook of Small Animal Therapeutics. New York, Churchill Livingstone, 1985, pp 127–148.

Kemppainen, R.J.: Principles of glucocorticoid therapy in nonendocrine diseases. *In* Kirk, R.W. (ed): Current Veterinary Therapy IX. Philadelphia, W.B. Saunders Company, 1986, pp 954–962.

Lloyd, D.: Investigation of effects of essential fatty acid supplementation in atopic dogs. Presented at the Congress of the Dermatology Study Group, British Society of Veterinary Dermatologists, London, April 2, 1987.

Lloyd, D.: The role of essential fatty acids in veterinary dermatology: A review of the mechanisms of action and results of clinical trials. Presented at the Annual Meeting of the American College of Veterinary Dermatology. Washington, D.C., April 15, 1988.

Miller, W.H., Griffin, C.E., et al: Clinical trial of DVM Derm Caps in the treatment of allergic diseases in dogs: A nonblinded study. J Am Anim Hosp Assoc (accepted for publication 1987).

Miller, W.H.: Nonsteroidal anti-inflammatory agents in the management of canine and feline pruritus. *In* Kirk, R.W. (ed): Current Veterinary Therapy X. Philadelphia, W.B. Saunders Company (in press).

Muller, G.H., Kirk, R.W., and Scott, D.W.: Small Animal Dermatology (ed 3). Philadelphia, W.B. Saunders Company, 1983, pp 167–174.

Mulnix, J.A.: Endocrine disorders. *In* Davis, L.E. (ed): Handbook of Small Animal Therapeutics. New York, Churchill Livingstone, 1985, pp 577–603.

Rosenthal, R.C., and Wilcke, J.R.: Glucocorticoid therapy. *In* Kirk, R.W. (ed): Current Veterinary Therapy VIII. Philadelphia, W.B. Saunders Company, 1983, pp 854–863.

Scott, D.W., and Buerger, R.G.: Nonsteroidal anti-inflammatory agents in the management of canine pruritus. J Am Anim Hosp Assoc 24:425–428, 1988.

Voith, V.L.: Behavioral disorders. *In* Davis, L.E. (ed): Handbook of Small Animal Therapeutics. New York, Churchill Livingstone, 1985, pp 519–548.

CHAPTER 7

Aas, K.: The critical approach to food allergy. Ann Allergy 51:256–259, 1983.

American Academy of Allergy and Immunology Committee on Adverse Reactions to Foods: Adverse Reactions to Foods. US Department of Health and Human Services, NIH Publication #84–2442, 1984.

Atkins, F.M., and Metcalf, D.D.: Diagnostic approaches to food allergy. Immunol Allergy Pract 71:37–43, 1983.

August, J.R.: Dietary hypersensitivity in dogs: Cutaneous manifestations, diagnosis, and management. Comp Cont Ed 7:469–480, 1985.

Baker, E.: Food allergy. Vet Clin North Am 4:79–89, 1974.

Haddad, Z.H.: Clinical and immunological aspects of food hypersensitivity. Ann Allergy 49:29–34, 1982.

Hannuksela, M.: Food allergy and skin diseases. Ann Allergy 51:269–272, 1983.

Lehman, C.W.: The leukocytic food allergy test: A study of its reliability and reproducibility. Effect of diet and sublingual food drops on this test. Ann Allergy 45:150–158, 1980.

McDougal, B.J.: Correlation of results of the radioallergosorbent test and provocative testing in 20 dogs with food allergy. Proceedings of the Annual AAVD and ACVD, 1987, p 42.

Muller, G.H., Kirk, R. W., and Scott, D.W.: Small Animal Dermatology (ed 3). Philadelphia, W.B. Saunders Company, 1983, pp 420–425.

Scott, D.W.: Immunologic skin disorders in the dog and cat. Vet Clin North Am 8:641–664, 1978.

Walton, G.S.: Skin responses in the dog and cat to ingested allergens. Observations on 100 confirmed cases. Vet Rec 81:709–713, 1967.

White, S.D.: Food hypersensitivity in 30 dogs. J Am Vet Med Assoc 188:695–698, 1986.

CHAPTER 8

Chamberlain, K.W.: Allergic contact dermatitis. Vet Clin North Am 4:147–152, 1974.

Graafar, S.M., and Krawiec, D.R.: Chemical sensitizers and contact dermatitis. J Am Anim Hosp Assoc 10:133, 1974.

Grant, D.I., and Thoday, K.L.: Canine allergic contact dermatitis: A clinical review. J Small Anim Pract 21:17–27, 1980.

Krawiec, D.R., and Graafar, S.M.: A comparative study of allergic and primary irritant contact dermatitis with dinitrochlorobenzene (DNCB) in dogs. J Invest Dermatol 65:248–251, 1975.

Kunkle, G.A., and Gross, T.L.: Allergic contact dermatitis to *Tradescantia fluminensis* (Wandering Jew) in a dog. Comp Cont Ed 5:925–930, 1983.

Maibach, H.I., and Epstein, E.: Contact dermatitis. *In* Middleton, E., Reed, C.E., and Ellis, E.F. (eds): Allergy: Principles and Practice (ed 2). St. Louis, C.V. Mosby Company, 1983, pp 1055–1079.

Muller, G.H., Kirk, R.W., and Scott, D.W.: Small Animal Dermatology (ed 3). Philadelphia, W.B. Saunders Company, 1983, pp 415–420.

Nesbitt, G.H., and Schmitz, J.A.: Contact dermatitis in the dog: A review of 35 cases. J Am Anim Hosp Assoc 13:155–163, 1977.

Ripps, J.H.: Allergic dermatitis in a dog. J Am Vet Med Assoc 133:479, 1958.

Slavin, R.G.: Allergic contact dermatitis. *In* Patterson, R. (ed): Allergic Disease: Diagnosis and Management (ed 2). Philadelphia, J.B. Lippincott Company, 1980, pp 584–598.

Walton, G.S.: Allergic contact dermatitis. *In* Kirk, R.W. (ed): Current Veterinary Therapy VI. Philadelphia, W.B. Saunders Company, 1977, pp 571–575.

CHAPTER 9

Georgi, J.R.: Parasitology for Veterinarians (ed 4). Philadelphia, W.B. Saunders Company, 1985, pp 30–34.

Halliwell, R.E.W.: Hyposensitization in the treatment of flea-bite hypersensitivity: Results of a double-blind study. J Am Anim Hosp Assoc 117:249–253, 1981.

Halliwell, R.E.W.: Factors in the development of flea-bite allergy. Vet Med 79:1273–1278, 1984.

Halliwell, R.E.W., and Schemmer, K.R.: The role of basophils in the immunopathogenesis of canine flea allergy dermatitis. Proceedings of the Annual AAVD and ACVD, 1985.

Halliwell, R.E.W.: Flea allergy: Pathogenesis, therapy, and flea control. Proceedings of the 52nd Annual Meeting of the American Animal Hospital Association, 1985, pp 145–149.

Kunkle, G.A., and Milcarsky, J.: Double-blind flea hyposensitization trial in cats. J Am Vet Med Assoc 186:677–680, 1985.

MacDonald, J.M., and Miller, T.A.: Parasiticide therapy in small animal dermatology. *In* Kirk, R.W. (ed): Current Veterinary Therapy IX. Philadelphia, W.B. Saunders Company, 1986, pp 571–590.

Melman, S.A., and Hutton, P.: Flea control on dogs and cats, indoors and in the environment. Comp Cont Ed 7:869–887, 1985.

Muller, G.H., Kirk, R.W., and Scott, D.W.: Small Animal Dermatology (ed 3). Philadelphia, W.B. Saunders Company, 1983, pp 432–439.

Schick, M.P., and Schick, R.O.: Understanding and implementing safe and effective flea control. J Am Anim Hosp Assoc 22:421–424, 1986.

Soulsby, E.J.L.: Helminths, Arthropods, and Protozoa of Domesticated Animals (ed 7). Philadelphia, Lea and Febiger, 1982, pp 378–384.

Van Winkle, K.A.: An evaluation of flea antigens used in intradermal skin testing for flea allergy in the canine. J Am Anim Hosp Assoc 17:343–354, 1981.

CHAPTER 10

Baker, B.B., and Stannard, A.A.: A look at canine scabies. J Am Anim Hosp Assoc 10:513–514, 1974.

Baker, B.B., and Stannard, A.A.: Drug eruption in a dog. J Am Vet Med Assoc 166:500–501, 1975.

Baker, E.: Staphylococcal disease. Vet Clin North Am 4:107–117, 1974.

Breen, P.T.: Secondary bacterial hypersensitivity reactions in canine skin. Proceedings of the 43rd Annual Meeting of the American Animal Hospital Association, 1976, pp 134–135.

Butler, J.M., Peters, J.E., et al: Pruritic dermatitis in asthmatic Basenji-Greyhound dogs: A model for human atopic dermatitis. J Am Acad Dermatol 8:33–38, 1983.

Fellner, M.J.: Drug reactions. *In* Stone, J. (ed): Dermatologic Immunology and Allergy. St. Louis, C.V. Mosby Company, 1985, pp 677–688.

Hirshman, C.A., Downes, H., et al: Basenji-Greyhound dog model of asthma: Pulmonary responses after beta-adrenergic blockage. J Appl Physiol 51:1423–1427, 1981.

Miller, T.A.: Immunology in intestinal parasitism. Vet Clin North Am 8:707–720, 1978.

Muller, G.H., Kirk, R.W., and Scott, D.W.: Small Animal Dermatology (ed 3). Philadelphia, W.B. Saunders Company, 1983, pp 163–164, 425–429, 440–448.

Halliwell, R.E.W.: The site of production and localization of IgE in canine tissues. Ann NY Acad Sci 254:476–488, 1975.

Powell, M.B., Weisbroth, S.H., et al: Reaginic hypersensitivity in *Otodectes cynotis* infection of cats and mode of mite feeding. Am J Vet Res 41:877–882, 1980.

Pukay, B.P.: Treatment of canine bacterial hypersensitivity by hyposensitization with *Staphylococcus aureus* bacterin-toxoid. J Am Anim Hosp Assoc 21:479–483, 1985.

Scott, D.W., MacDonald, J.M., and Schultz, R.D.: Staphylococcal hypersensitivity in the dog. J Am Anim Hosp Assoc 13:766–779, 1978.

Scott, D.W.: Drug eruptions. *In* Kirk, R.W. (ed): Current Veterinary Therapy VII. Philadelphia, W.B. Saunders Company, 1980, pp 458–461.

Solomon, W.R., and Mathews, K.P.: Serobiology and inhalant allergens. *In* Middleton, E., Reed, C.E., and Ellis, E.F. (eds): Allergy Principles and Practice. St. Louis, C.V. Mosby Company, 1978, pp 899–956.

Vollset, I.: Immediate type hypersensitivity in dogs induced by storage mites. Res Vet Sci 40:123–127, 1986.

Walton, G.S.: Symposium on allergic and endocrine dermatoses in the dog and cat. I. Allergic dermatoses of the dog and cat. J Small Anim Pract 7:749–754, 1966.

Wintroub, B.V., Shiffman, N.J., and Arndt, K.A.: Adverse cutaneous reactions to drugs. *In* Fitzpatrick, T.B., Eisen, A.Z., Wolff, K., et al (eds): Dermatology in General Medicine (ed 2). New York, McGraw-Hill, 1979, pp 555–567.

Witkowski, J.A., and Parish, L.C.: Immunology of scabies and pediculosis. *In* Stone, J. (ed): Dermatologic Immunology and Allergy. St. Louis, C.V. Mosby Company, 1985, pp 707–709.

Index

Note: The letter i following a page number refers to an illustration; the letter t following a page number refers to a table.